Interdisciplinary Rheumatology
Rheumatology and Cardiology

A key problem in medicine is that certain diseases may involve organ systems that cross the boundaries of individual specialties. For instance, a patient with scleroderma can develop myocarditis, or one with vasculitis can manifest with aortitis, which in turn can affect the function of the aortic valve. This book represents a dialogue between specialties, helping clinicians understand the implications of disease both within their own specialty and in the overlapping specialty of the case. Here, leading experts from the fields of rheumatology and cardiology provide a masterclass in the care of patients with systemic illnesses that involve the immune system and the cardiovascular system.

Key Features:

- Provides a clinical approach to the patient with cardiovascular manifestations of rheumatic disease
- Details cutting-edge research with inputs from the world's leading experts
- Discusses possible future directions for research and advancement

Interdisciplinary Rheumatology Series

Rheumatology and Gastroenterology
Edited by Reem Jan and Sushila Dalal

Rheumatology and Cardiology
Edited by Vaneet K Sandhu

For more information on this series, please visit https://www.routledge.com/
Interdisciplinary-Rheumatology/book-series/IRJL

Interdisciplinary Rheumatology
Rheumatology and Cardiology

Edited by
Vaneet K. Sandhu, MD, MS, RhMSUS, FACR

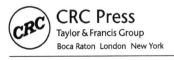

CRC Press
Taylor & Francis Group
Boca Raton London New York

CRC Press is an imprint of the
Taylor & Francis Group, an **informa** business

First edition published 2025
by CRC Press
2385 NW Executive Center Drive, Suite 320, Boca Raton FL 33431

and by CRC Press
4 Park Square, Milton Park, Abingdon, Oxon, OX14 4RN

CRC Press is an imprint of Taylor & Francis Group, LLC

ISBN: 978-1-032-47953-8 (hbk)
ISBN: 978-1-032-47221-8 (pbk)
ISBN: 978-1-003-38671-1 (ebk)

DOI: 10.1201/9781003386711

Typeset in Minion Pro
by KnowledgeWorks Global Ltd.

Dedication

To my husband, Gary, and children, Sayva and Sehj, whose love and support fuel my ambitions and growth. To my mentors and colleagues who have inspired me. And to my patients, who have taught me more than any textbook ever could.

Contents

About the Editor

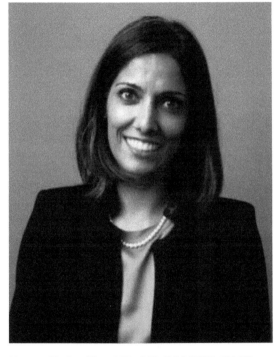

Vaneet K. Sandhu, MD, MS, RhMSUS, FACR

Dr. Sandhu is the Vice President for Clinical Development, heading Autoimmunity with Fate Therapeutics Inc. and former Associate Professor of Medicine in the Division of Rheumatology at Loma Linda University Health (LLUH). She began her medical journey in India, followed by internal medicine residency at Loma Linda University Health. She completed her rheumatology fellowship at Cedars-Sinai Medical Center in Los Angeles, California. Recognizing the crucial role of education in fostering excellence in healthcare, Dr. Sandhu pursued and earned a Master of Science in Academic Medicine, which was instrumental in her role as the rheumatology fellowship program director at LLUH, where she passionately contributed to shaping the next generation of rheumatologists.

Beyond clinical and educational roles, Dr. Sandhu has served on various committees with the American College of Rheumatology. Her recent work on the Committee on Training and Workforce Issues in addition to the Collaborative Initiatives Network allowed her to play a vital role in providing patient education resources and supporting the growth of trainees in the field. Additionally, as a chapter leader for the Association of Women in Rheumatology, she has coordinated collaborative educational events, fostering a sense of community and shared learning within the rheumatology field.

Dr. Sandhu's research endeavors have focused on critical areas such as healthcare disparities, medical education, and lupus. Her commitment to advancing knowledge in these domains is evident through her numerous publications as well as funded research studies, which have contributed significantly to the scholarly landscape of rheumatology.

Contributors

Nasam Alfraji MD
Division of Rheumatology, Loma Linda University
Medical Center, Loma Linda, California, USA

In Hae Baek MD
Department of Medicine, Loma Linda University
Health, Loma Linda, California, USA

Gizem Bilgili MD
Smidt Heart Institute, Cedars-Sinai Medical
Center, Los Angeles, California, USA

Marven Gerel Cabling MD
Division of Rheumatology, Loma Linda University
Medical Center, Loma Linda, California, USA

Kathleena D'Anna
Division of Rheumatology, Loma Linda University
Health, Loma Linda, California, USA

Alaa Diab MD
Department of Internal Medicine, Greater
Baltimore Medical Center, Towson, Maryland,
USA; Johns Hopkins Bloomberg School of Public
Health, Baltimore, Maryland, USA

Loomee Doo MD
Department of Rheumatology, Veterans Affairs
Loma Linda Healthcare System, Loma Linda,
California, USA

Christina Downey MD
Division of Rheumatology, Loma Linda University
Health, Loma Linda, California, USA

Anisha B. Dua MD, MPH
Division of Rheumatology, Northwestern
University Feinberg School of Medicine, Chicago,
Illinois, USA

Heather Gillespie
Division of Rheumatology, Loma Linda University
Health, Loma Linda, California, USA

Alpha Shanika Gonzalez FNP-BC
Division of Rheumatology, Department
of Medicine, Loma Linda University School
of Medicine, Loma Linda, California, USA

Martha Gulati MD MS FACC FAHA FASPC FESC
Barbra Streisand Women's Heart Center,
Smidt Heart Institute, Cedars-Sinai Medical
Center, Los Angeles, California, USA

Breanna Hansen MD
Department of Internal Medicine, Cedars-
Sinai Medical Center, Los Angeles,
California, USA

Christopher Hino
Department of Internal Medicine, Loma
Linda University Medical Center, Loma Linda,
California, USA

Jessica N. Holtzman
Division of Cardiology, University of California,
San Francisco, California, USA

Brian D. Jaros MD
Division of Rheumatology, Northwestern
University Feinberg School of Medicine, Chicago,
Illinois, USA

Muhammad U. Javaid DO
Division of Rheumatology, Medical College of
Georgia at Augusta University, Augusta, Georgia,
USA

Talha Khawar MD
Division of Rheumatology, Loma Linda University
Health; VA Loma Linda Medical Center, Loma
Linda, California, USA

C. Kent Kwoh MD
Division of Rheumatology, University of Arizona
Arthritis Center, Arizona, USA

Sophia Li MD
University of California Riverside School of Medicine, Riverside, California, USA; Loma Linda University School of Medicine, Loma Linda, California, USA

Ryan Massay MBBS (HONS)
University of Michigan, Ann Arbor, Michigan, USA

C. Noel Bairey Merz MD
Barbra Streisand Women's Heart Center, Smidt Heart Institute, Cedars-Sinai Medical Center, Los Angeles, California, USA

Artem Minalyan MD
Division of Rheumatology, Loma Linda University Health, Loma Linda, California, USA

Noelle A. Rolle MBBS, FACR
Division of Rheumatology, Department of Medicine, Medical College of Georgia at Augusta University; Augusta, Georgia, USA

Dana Song
Department of Pediatrics, Loma Linda University Children's Hospital, Loma Linda, California, USA

Karina D. Torralba MD FACR, MACM, CCD, CPI, RHMSUS
Division of Rheumatology, Department of Medicine, Loma Linda University School of Medicine, Loma Linda, California, USA; University of California Riverside School of Medicine, Riverside, California, USA

Diana H. Tran
Department of Internal Medicine, Cedars-Sinai Medical Center, Los Angeles, California, USA

Janet Wei MD
Barbra Streisand Women's Heart Center, Smidt Heart Institute, Cedars-Sinai Medical Center, Los Angeles, California, USA

Diana Yang MD
Department of Medicine; Division of Rheumatology, Loma Linda University Health, Loma Linda, California, USA

Approach to the patient with cardiac manifestations of rheumatic disease

TALHA KHAWAR AND IN HAE BAEK

INTRODUCTION

Systemic autoimmune diseases are characterized by abnormal activation of the immune system autoreactive to self-tissues and antigens. These diseases bear a significant burden on the cardiovascular system by way of causing premature coronary artery disease, vasculitis, pericarditis, myocarditis, endocarditis, conduction system abnormalities as well as structural abnormalities of the heart valves.[1] For this reason, it is imperative to recognize these cardiovascular effects early in the disease course and to initiate prompt, appropriate treatment to minimize end-organ damage and mortality. Since some of these effects can be subclinical and may not be overtly evident at initial evaluation, it is critical to have a high level of suspicion for cardiac involvement when evaluating a patient with rheumatic disease.

PERICARDITIS AND PERICARDIAL INVOLVEMENT

Pericardial involvement is most frequently observed in systemic lupus erythematosus (SLE), with up to 54% of patients experiencing a pericardial effusion during their disease course. It is also frequently seen in patients with rheumatoid arthritis, scleroderma, and Sjogren's syndrome.[2]

Acute pericarditis usually presents as acute pleuritic chest pain with a sudden onset of symptoms. Chest pain improves with leaning forward or sitting upright and worsens with lying supine.[3] Physical examination is usually significant for a pericardial friction rub, which is a coarse sound heard during auscultation at the left sternal border. Though this is pathognomonic for pericarditis, it may not be present in up to two thirds of patients. Electrocardiogram (ECG) typically shows ST segment elevations in all limb leads and chest leads in these patients. PR segment depression is also a feature seen in up to 60% of younger patients with acute pericarditis (Figure 1.1).[4] ST segment elevation is global, which is different from acute myocardial infarction where ST segment elevation is usually localized to the affected segment. The ST segment elevations usually resolve within a few days followed by T-wave inversions. Subacute or chronic pericarditis may have a slightly varied presentation. The presence of leukocytosis on complete blood count and elevated inflammatory markers such as erythrocyte sedimentation rate (ESR) and C-reactive protein (CRP) is also typically seen in these patients.[4]

The presence of cardiomegaly on a chest radiograph is usually suggestive of a large pericardial effusion, which can lead to cardiac tamponade. Echocardiography, either transthoracic or transesophageal, tends to have a better sensitivity for evaluating smaller pericardial effusions.[5] Late gadolinium enhancement of the pericardium on cardiac MRI is highly associated with pericarditis on histopathology and is also used in clinical practice for establishing a diagnosis of acute or

DOI: 10.1201/9781003386711-1

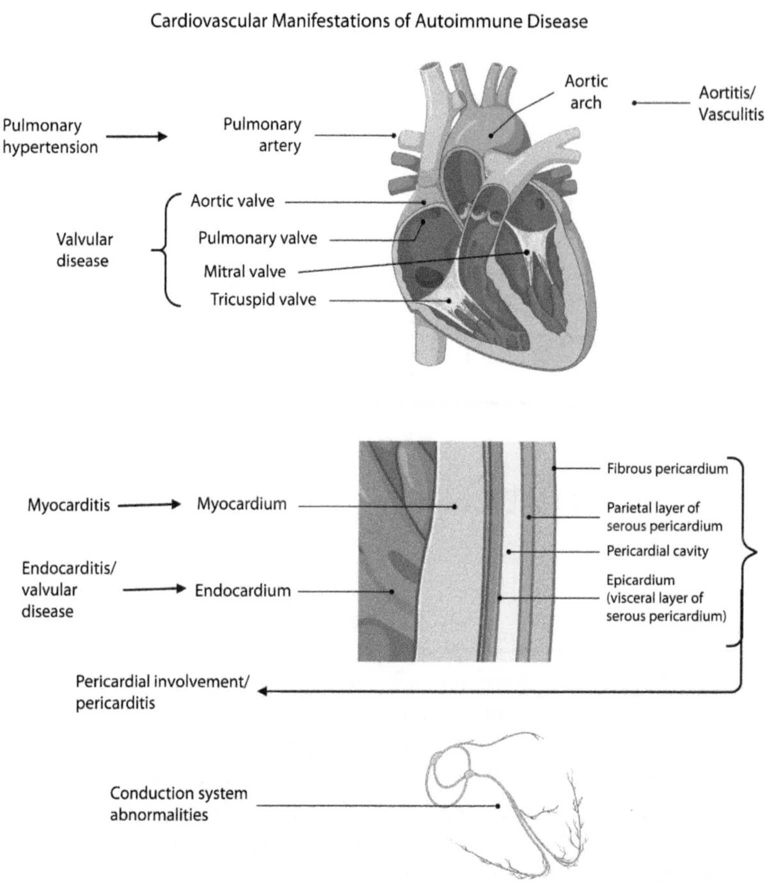

Cardiovascular Manifestations of Autoimmune Disease
Pulmonary hypertension
Pulmonary artery
Aortic arch
Aortitis/ Vasculitis
Valvular disease
Aortic valve
Pulmonary valve
Mitral valve
Tricuspid valve
Myocarditis
Myocardium
Endocarditis/ valvular disease
Endocardium
Fibrous pericardium
Parietal layer of serous pericardium
Pericardial cavity
Epicardium (visceral layer of serous pericardium)
Pericardial involvement/ pericarditis
Conduction system abnormalities

Figure 1.A Illustration showing various regions of the heart affected by rheumatologic conditions.

I
aVR
V1
V4
II
aVL
V2
V5
III
aVF
V3
V6
V1
II
V5

ST segment elevation: red arrows
PR segment depression: blue arrows

Figure 1.1 EKG changes typically seen in acute pericarditis include global ST segment elevation and corresponding PR segment depression.

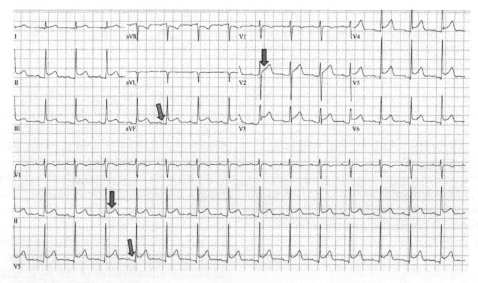

Table 1.1 Diagnosis and management of pericardial disease

Acute pericarditis	Pericarditis can be diagnosed with at least two of the following four criteria:
	• Pericardiac/pleuritic chest pain • Pericardial rub • New widespread ST elevation or PR depression on ECG • Pericardial effusion (new or worsening)
	Additional supporting findings: Elevated ESR, CRP, white blood cell count, and evidence of pericardial inflammation by imaging (CT, CMR, and ECHO)
Recurrent pericarditis	Recurrence of pericarditis after documented evidence of first episode of acute pericarditis and a symptom-free interval of 4–6 weeks or longer
Incessant pericarditis	Pericarditis lasting for > 4–6 weeks but < 3 months without remission
Chronic pericarditis	Pericarditis lasting > 3 months

Source: Adapted from Adler et al. [7]

recurrent pericarditis. Cardiac MRI is also used to clinically follow such patients for treatment response.[6] Elevated ESR and CRP, though non-specific, are also reported in patients with acute pericarditis. Patients with concomitant myocardial involvement may also present with elevated cardiac enzymes such as creatine phosphokinase (CPK) as well as troponins. Diagnosis of acute and recurrent pericarditis can be made using proposed diagnostic criteria by the European Society of Cardiology (ESC) Task Force for the Diagnosis and Management of Pericardial Diseases (Table 1.1).[7]

Once the diagnosis of acute pericarditis has been established, prompt medical management is critical.[8] The ESC recommends stratifying patients with acute pericarditis symptoms into high-risk and low-risk groups based on their presentations. Patients with major poor prognostic factors such as fever of more than 38°C (100.4°F), subacute onset, large pericardial effusion, cardiac tamponade, or lack of response to aspirin or nonsteroidal anti-inflammatory drugs (NSAIDs) after 1 week of therapy should be considered for hospitalization (Table 1.2). In addition, patients who are on immunosuppressants, have a history of trauma, or are on anticoagulation therapy should also be considered for treatment in a hospital setting. Patients who do not have these risk factors can be managed as outpatients.[7]

Treatment of pericardial disease

NSAIDs are considered first-line therapy for treatment of acute pericarditis and for the treatment of acute recurrences (Figure 1.2). High doses of NSAIDs are associated with increased risk for gastric ulcers, gastrointestinal bleeding, and renal failure. Colchicine has been used as first-line therapy for treatment of acute pericarditis either alone or in combination with NSAIDs. This combination is also employed for treatment of acute recurrences in patients with history of previously treated pericarditis. Colchicine has also shown benefits in preventing recurrence in patients with their first episode of pericarditis.[9,10] The most common side effect associated with colchicine is gastrointestinal disturbance, including diarrhea. It may also be associated with bone marrow suppression and myopathy.

Corticosteroids have also been used mostly as a second- or third-line treatment option for patients with acute pericarditis. It is important to note that use of corticosteroids has been associated with an increased risk for recurrence in these patients. Therefore, it is recommended to use a low-dose

Table 1.2 Predictors of poor outcomes in pericarditis

Major predictors	Minor predictors
Fever > 38°C	Myopericarditis
Subacute onset	Immunosuppression
Large pericardial effusion	Trauma
Cardiac tamponade	Oral anticoagulant therapy
Lack of response to aspirin or NSAIDs within 1 week of treatment	

Source: Adapted from Adler et al. [7]

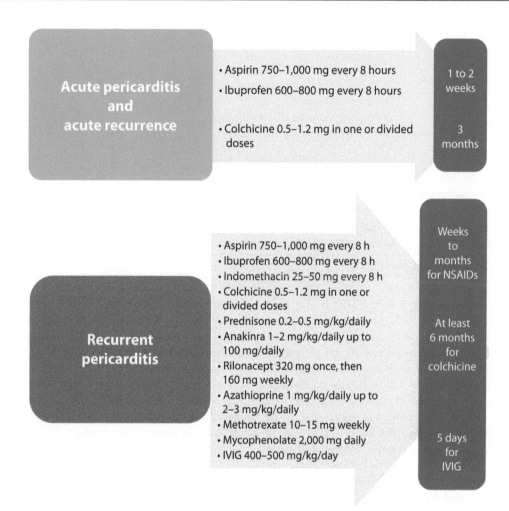

Figure 1.2 Pharmacologic treatments suggested for acute and recurrent pericarditis.

(0.2 mg/kg/day to 0.5 mg/kg/day) prednisone equivalent of corticosteroids for the treatment of patients who have either failed initial treatment with NSAIDs and colchicine or are not candidates for those treatments.[3,11]

Interleukin-1 (IL-1) inhibition was also used successfully in randomized clinical trials for patients with recurrence as well as initial therapy for acute pericarditis. The use of anakinra, an IL-1α and IL-1β antagonist, for the treatment of pericarditis has demonstrated efficacy in both reducing the dose of corticosteroids and improving pain and inflammatory markers in these patients. Daily subcutaneous injections with anakinra, however, can be bothersome for some patients, and injection site reactions have been frequently reported.[12,13] Canakinumab, an intravenous IL-1β antagonist, has also demonstrated benefit in pericarditis patients with underlying adult-onset Still's disease,

but its use in the setting of other systemic autoimmune diseases remains to be validated.[14]

Other immunosuppressive or immune-modulatory agents such as azathioprine, mycophenolate, and methotrexate, as well as intravenous immunoglobulin (IVIG) treatment, have also been studied in the treatment of pericarditis in systemic rheumatic disease with demonstrated benefit as steroid-sparing agents. The presence of specific underlying autoimmune disease can help direct the use of these medications for individual patients.[3]

Creating a pericardial window or conducting a pericardiectomy is considered in patients with cardiac tamponade or refractory disease. The ESC recommends avoiding strenuous activity until CRP has normalized in patients who are not participating in competitive sports. Patients who participate in competitive sports should wait until diagnostic tests such as ECG and echocardiogram have normalized prior to participating in competitive sports. Some experts believe at least 3 months of rest from competitive sports is necessary to prevent complications.[7]

CORONARY ARTERY DISEASE

Coronary artery disease is more prevalent in patients with systemic autoimmune rheumatic diseases such as SLE, rheumatoid arthritis, psoriatic arthritis, and spondyloarthropathies compared to age-matched controls. In individuals with SLE, the prevalence of coronary artery disease increases with advancing age, and it stands as the primary risk factor leading to death in 33% of these patients.[15,16] Despite taking into consideration traditional risk factors such as hyperlipidemia, diabetes, hypertension, and obesity, patients with systemic autoimmune diseases tend to have a higher risk of coronary artery disease compared to age-matched controls. Chronic inflammation and cytokine-induced vascular damage leading to atherosclerosis are significant risk factors in these patients.[17] The use of immunomodulatory agents such as glucocorticoids may also contribute to accelerated coronary artery disease in such patients.[18]

Symptoms of acute coronary syndrome (ACS) tend to be similar in patients with and without systemic autoimmune disease. Patients with systemic autoimmune diseases, such as rheumatoid arthritis, often underreport symptoms of angina, leading to an underrecognized burden of coronary artery disease.[19] Patients with SLE can experience atypical symptoms such as dyspnea and diaphoresis, which may go unrecognized as related to underlying coronary artery disease.

The European League Against Rheumatism (EULAR) recommends applying general cardiovascular risk stratification guidance for patients with Sjogren's syndrome, rheumatoid arthritis, gout, systemic sclerosis, and myositis.[20] Some of the most notable risk stratification tools include the Framingham risk score (FRS), QRISK3, and Systemic COronary Risk Evaluation (SCORE). While the group did not report any benefit of using low-dose aspirin or other antiplatelet therapies for prophylaxis in most of these patients, special attention is necessary for patients with ANCA-associated vasculitis and SLE when using risk stratification. There is data to suggest that these tools may underestimate the presence of cardiovascular disease in SLE and ANCA-associated vasculitis. Particularly, the FRS underestimates the

coronary artery disease risk in women, who make up the majority of patients with SLE.[20]

Work from the Hopkins lupus cohort showed that in addition to traditional risk factors, the presence of low serum complement C3, positive lupus anticoagulant (LAC), and high disease activity scores portend an increased risk of cardiovascular events in SLE patients.[21]

There are currently no specific biomarkers used in patients with systemic autoimmune diseases to diagnose the presence of coronary artery disease. Elevated CRP and serum homocysteine levels can be helpful, though they are not routinely used in clinical practice for this purpose. Coronary computed tomography (CT) angiography has been utilized in patients with SLE to reveal the presence of early coronary artery disease. The capability to detect coronary artery disease in asymptomatic SLE patients, which is not observed in controls, establishes CT angiography as a potential tool in risk assessment for patients with SLE. It can be employed in clinical practice for early identification and management of cardiovascular issues in this population.[22,23]

In addition to managing traditional risk factors, the EULAR recommends maintaining a blood pressure target of < 130/80 mmHg in all SLE patients. The use of ACE inhibitors and angiotensin receptor blockers (ARBs) is recommended in patients with lupus nephritis who have arterial hypertension or a urine protein-to-creatinine ratio of more than 500 mg/g/day. The use of antiplatelet agents needs to be individualized in patients with antiphospholipid syndrome (APS) and SLE. A high-risk antiphospholipid antibody profile should prompt the use of low-dose aspirin or other antiplatelet therapy in both primary APS patients and patients with SLE. This includes individuals with a positive serum LAC, triple-positive antiphospholipid antibody testing (LAC + anti-cardiolipin antibody + anti-ß$_2$Glycoprotein-1 antibody), or isolated persistently positive anti-cardiolipin antibody (aCL) at medium to high titers. As in other systemic autoimmune diseases mentioned above, lipid profile management in patients with SLE and APS should be based on general population guidelines.

There is robust data in favor of using hydroxychloroquine to reduce cardiovascular events in patients with SLE. EULAR recommends the routine use of hydroxychloroquine in all patients with SLE to help reduce their cardiovascular risk unless there are strong contraindications against the use of hydroxychloroquine.[20]

CONDUCTION SYSTEM ABNORMALITIES

Conduction system abnormalities are seen frequently in patients with systemic and cardiac sarcoidosis, typically presenting as atrioventricular (AV) block and ventricular arrhythmias. While atrial involvement is less common than ventricular involvement, it can lead to cardiomyopathy, resulting in high morbidity in these patients. Therefore, it is crucial to screen all sarcoidosis patients experiencing symptoms such as palpitations, chest pain, a history of syncope, presyncope, abnormal ECG, abnormal Holter cardiac monitoring, and abnormal echocardiography for cardiac sarcoidosis. Palpitations are considered clinically relevant when the patient has experienced those symptoms for more than 2 weeks. An abnormal ECG is defined as complete left or right bundle branch block (BBB) and/or the presence of unexplained pathological Q waves in 2 or more leads and/or sustained second- or third-degree AV block and/or sustained or non-sustained ventricular tachycardia (VT). An abnormal echocardiogram is defined as regional wall motion abnormality and/or wall aneurysm and/or basal septum thinning and/or left ventricular ejection fraction (LVEF) < 40%. The Heart Rhythm Society (HRS) has published a consensus statement and guidelines for screening patients with systemic sarcoidosis for cardiac involvement, and a suggested algorithm for screening patients with biopsy-proven sarcoidosis for cardiac involvement is shown in Figure 1.3.[24]

Cardiac conduction system abnormalities are also commonly reported in patients with systemic sclerosis. This is thought to be due to fibrosis of the conduction system with or without underlying myocardial fibrosis, mostly in the setting of vascular compromise. Patients with early conduction system abnormalities such as first-degree AV block or isolated BBB may be asymptomatic. More advanced conduction system abnormalities, such as second- or third-degree AV blocks, can lead to symptoms like fatigue, exercise intolerance, presyncope, and syncope.[25] The UK systemic sclerosis working group recommends performing an ECG in all patients with a new diagnosis of systemic sclerosis. In cases where there is clinical suspicion for conduction system abnormalities, a Holter monitor or event monitor should also be considered. Treatments commonly used in the general

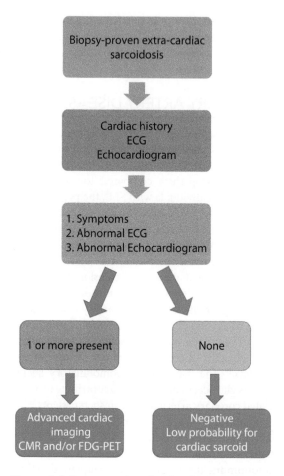

Figure 1.3 Suggested evaluation for a patient with biopsy-proven extra-cardiac sarcoidosis.

population for specific arrhythmias, including the use of antiarrhythmic medications and cardiac ablation therapy, may also be applied to patients with systemic sclerosis for similar indications.[26]

Atrial fibrillation and associated stroke were reported to be higher in patients with rheumatoid arthritis, according to a long-term cohort study conducted in Denmark, although other studies have not conclusively associated rheumatoid arthritis with atrial fibrillation.[27]

Conduction system abnormalities have also been reported in patients with SLE. An international cohort study showed that almost 30% of asymptomatic patients with SLE have nonspecific ST–T-segment abnormalities on ECG, and nearly 15% of patients had a prolonged QT interval. A prolonged QT interval has been demonstrated as an independent risk factor for cardiovascular mortality in the general population, likely due to its contribution to ventricular arrhythmia and sudden cardiac death.[28] In patients with SLE, this is clinically significant, as most of these patients are on or need to be on hydroxychloroquine for treatment of SLE, which is well-known to cause prolongation of the QT interval. It might be helpful to perform a baseline ECG in patients with SLE who are starting hydroxychloroquine to identify any underlying prolonged QT interval. Medication interaction should also be considered when evaluating such patients, as concomitant use of QT-prolonging medications with hydroxychloroquine may worsen the underlying conduction abnormality and increase the risk for ventricular arrhythmias.

MYOCARDITIS

Myocarditis is an inflammatory condition that involves the cardiac myocardium, often seen in association with the involvement of the conduction system of the heart, as well as the pericardium. This inflammation results in a vast array of symptoms ranging from asymptomatic myocarditis discovered by cardiac magnetic resonance (CMR) imaging to arrhythmias, dilated cardiomyopathy, and even sudden cardiac death. Myocarditis is considered one of the secondary cardiomyopathies that can lead to structural damage to the cardiac tissue.[29]

Myocarditis can be caused by infectious and non-infectious conditions. Infectious causes include, but are not limited to, coxsackievirus, adenovirus, coronaviruses, including COVID-19, influenza, *Trypanosoma cruzi*, *Borrelia*, and HIV, among others. Drugs like clozapine, immune checkpoint inhibitors, and tricyclic antidepressants can also trigger myocarditis in addition to cardiotoxins such as cocaine, marijuana, and methamphetamines. Autoimmune diseases, exposure to radiation, and hypersensitivity reactions may trigger myocarditis, as well as mRNA vaccine- and smallpox vaccine-associated myocarditis.[30,31]

Some systemic autoimmune diseases known to cause myocarditis include SLE, sarcoidosis, ANCA-associated vasculitis, giant cell arteritis, Takayasu's arteritis, and idiopathic inflammatory myopathies. The prevalence of lupus myocarditis has been reported to be anywhere between 10 and 60% of patients with SLE.[32] Clinically observable myocarditis is seen in about 5% patients with systemic sarcoidosis; however, 20–25% of patients have asymptomatic cardiac involvement.[32,33] The

risk of SLE myocarditis is increased in patients with earlier onset of disease.[34]

As the pathogenesis of any autoimmune disease involves the deficit of self-regulation by the immune system and, therefore, an inappropriate response of the body to its native tissues and organs, the pathologic process of autoimmune myocarditis is similar. Unchecked immune system attacks and injures the myocytes. The lymphocytic predominance seen in autoimmune myocarditis suggests a T-cell-mediated pathophysiology. T-cell infiltration and cytokine production in the heart lead to muscle damage, remodeling, and myocyte death.[35]

Autoimmune myocarditis displays a wide range of clinical symptoms, from being asymptomatic, having dyspnea, to having chest pain, or even presenting with fulminant cardiogenic shock. Fever with chest pain is also reported in up to 65% patients. Asymptomatic, chronic myocarditis may progress to heart failure and dilated cardiomyopathy. In patients presenting with chest pain, ACS must be ruled out. Patients may also present with acute, new-onset heart failure, typically in the absence of traditional risk factors such as coronary artery disease, diabetes mellitus, and hypertension. Arrhythmias, both life-threatening and not, can also be the presenting symptom that prompts patients to seek medical attention. In any of these cases – chest pain, heart failure, cardiogenic shock, and arrhythmias – potentially life-threatening causes must be ruled out and addressed before investigating myocarditis as the potential underlying etiology.[36–38]

The diagnosis of autoimmune myocarditis depends on several factors. First, the clinical presentation, including medical history with the support of lab tests and imaging, is necessary to help establish the diagnosis. Clinical findings, however, as mentioned above, vary greatly and are often nonspecific. Also, unlike pericarditis, ECG findings in myocarditis, typically sinus tachycardia with ST segment changes, or T-wave inversions, are also nonspecific. ST segment elevations are seen in ACS and up to 80% of patients with acute myocarditis.[39] Echocardiogram in myocarditis will typically demonstrate wall motion abnormalities, particularly in the inferior and lateral walls.[29,37] There are also no specific laboratory findings in myocarditis. An elevation in troponins and creatine kinase MB (CK-MB) and inflammatory markers, like ESR and CRP, can help guide in diagnosis. In one study, elevated CRP was seen up to 80% of patients presenting with acute myocarditis and elevated high-sensitivity troponin as well as CPK was seen in up to 99% of these patients.[40] Elevated inflammatory markers and elevated CPK with troponin are nonspecific.

Viral antibody titers are rarely of any diagnostic significance except for HIV and Borrelia serologies, which, in the correct clinical context, can help narrow the diagnosis to those two infections. The presence of autoantibodies specific to systemic autoimmune diseases can be helpful in patients with a prior diagnosis of or high suspicion for systemic autoimmune disease. Peripheral eosinophilia noted on a complete blood count can point toward a diagnosis of eosinophilic myocarditis.[29]

Echocardiography is noninvasive, readily available, and routinely done in patients with suspected cardiac symptomatology. Acute myocarditis may present as segmental wall motion abnormalities (particularly in the inferior and inferior lateral walls), and abnormalities in right ventricular dysfunction, tissue Doppler imaging, and myocardial echogenicity. Early in the disease course, up to 75% of patients will retain normal left ventricular dimensions despite a severe reduction in the LVEF.[29]

The gold standard for diagnosing myocarditis is an endomyocardial biopsy (EMB). EMB is an invasive procedure that may lead to complications in up to 2% of the patients in expert centers and up to 8.9% of the patients in low volume centers with less expertise in this procedure. EMB also has low sensitivity which can result in underdiagnosis.[29,41,42]

CMR imaging with T2 mapping has been a preferred diagnostic modality due to its noninvasive nature and its ability to unveil silent myocarditis. CMR is also extremely helpful in the early diagnosis of myocarditis, regardless of the underlying cause. Therefore, CMR can be used with high diagnostic certainty when the diagnosis of myocarditis remains uncertain in patients.[43] The following three criteria are typically used in confirming the diagnosis of myocarditis while using CMR:

1. Increased regional or global myocardial signal intensity in T2-weighted images.
2. Increased global myocardial early gadolinium enhancement ratio between myocardium and skeletal muscle in gadolinium-enhanced T1-weighted images.
3. There is at least one focal lesion with non-ischemic regional distribution in inversion recovery-prepared gadolinium-enhanced T1-weighted images (also called late gadolinium enhancement).

The presence of two of the above three criteria is considered highly specific for the presence of myocarditis.[44] A possible limitation of using CMR arises in patients with severe left ventricular dysfunction, causing orthopnea and difficulty in lying supine for the scan. Additionally, patients with severe claustrophobia or those with cardiac pacemakers or defibrillators are not suitable candidates for CMR.

In cases where CMR is contraindicated, positron emission tomography (PET) can be utilized. PET scans are particularly useful for diagnosing and monitoring patients with cardiac sarcoidosis and those with systemic autoimmune diseases that may affect multiple organ systems.[45]

The management of acute autoimmune myocarditis follows a similar approach as non-autoimmune causes of myocarditis. The choice of therapies primarily depends on the severity of symptoms. It is crucial to address any life-threatening arrhythmias, such as ventricular fibrillation or high-grade AV blocks, before treating myocarditis.

Patients with acute myocarditis can be classified into two categories: Those with uncomplicated myocarditis and those with complicated disease. Complicated disease is characterized by left ventricular systolic dysfunction, acute heart failure, ventricular arrhythmias, advanced AV conduction abnormalities, or cardiogenic shock.

Patients with uncomplicated diseases can be managed with supportive care and monitoring. The use of NSAIDs, including aspirin, may be considered for symptom relief, though the evidence supporting the efficacy of NSAIDs in reducing inflammatory injury and improving left ventricular injection fracture is not necessarily significant.[46]

For patients with complicated diseases, a more aggressive management approach is warranted. The ESC Working Group on Myocardial and Pericardial Disease recommends the initial focus to be on stabilizing the patient's condition. In cases of acute heart failure, diuretics may be used to manage fluid overload. Arrhythmias, especially ventricular arrhythmias, may require antiarrhythmic medications or interventions. Athletes participating in competitive sports should avoid exercise for a minimum of 6 months after the initial episode.[37]

Therapy for autoimmune myocarditis typically involves use of corticosteroids as first-line treatment, followed by other immunosuppressive therapies used as steroid-sparing agents. Different combinations of corticosteroids, cyclosporine, and/or azathioprine have been the mainstays of treatment, though patients with SLE myocarditis have been treated successfully with cyclophosphamide as well.[35] For myocarditis associated with catastrophic APS (CAPS), treatment involves anticoagulation with vitamin K analogs, high-dose corticosteroids, and plasma exchange. In certain cases of CAPS myocarditis, Rituximab is used in combination with plasma exchange.[47] In some studies focusing on new-onset dilated cardiomyopathy secondary to myocarditis, high-dose IVIG administration has demonstrated improvement in LVEF.[48,49] Myocarditis associated with cardiac sarcoidosis is treated with corticosteroids as the first-line therapy, followed by methotrexate and anti-TNF inhibitors as second- and third-line therapies, respectively.[36] In cases where medical therapies do not yield positive responses, cardiac transplant may be considered.

VALVULAR DISEASE

Valvular disease occurs when any of the four heart valves do not function appropriately. It is typically characterized by the presence of vegetations, valve thickening, and valvular dysfunction.[50] This phenomenon is observed in certain types of autoimmune diseases, particularly in SLE and APS, where the risk of valvular disease is three times higher compared to other disorders such as rheumatoid arthritis.[51] Valvular disease can be asymptomatic, leading to severe cardiac dysfunction or even mortality due to its lack of early detection. Recognizing these cardiovascular effects early in the disease course and initiating appropriate management can minimize morbidity and mortality. Detecting valvular compromise requires a high level of suspicion, as patients with autoimmune diseases are more susceptible to valvular heart disease compared to those without immune dysfunction.[52]

Libman–Sacks endocarditis, or non-bacterial thrombotic endocarditis (NBTE), is a type of valvular disease characterized by the presence of sterile vegetations that typically form on the mitral, tricuspid, or aortic valves. These vegetations develop as a result of inflammation in conjunction with a hypercoagulable state and are frequently associated with SLE and APS. Underlying malignancy is observed in up to 59% patients with NBTE and should also be considered in these cases.[53] The presence of antiphospholipid antibodies is associated with a high prevalence of NBTE, and the presence of aCL increases this risk threefold in patients with SLE.[51] Nonspecific findings such as

thickened and calcified valves of endocarditis were found in 9–70% of autopsies in patients with rheumatoid arthritis, but these findings rarely exhibit any clinical symptoms in patients.[54] Aortic regurgitation, a form of valvular disease, is observed in various vasculitides, including Takayasu's arteritis, granulomatosis with polyangiitis, and Behçet syndrome. It is also commonly reported in sarcoidosis.[55] A population-based study indicated a fourfold increased risk of valvular heart disease in patients with systemic sclerosis compared to the general population.[56] Inflammation is the general, underlying pathogenesis of valvular defects in autoimmune diseases, though the specific processes leading to valvular dysfunction are disease dependent. In systemic sclerosis, the deposition of collagen fibers leads to valvular stenosis.[57]

The presentation of valvular disease due to autoimmune causes is not indistinguishable from other causes of valvular dysfunction. Most patients present with symptoms of shortness of breath, fatigue, chest pain, dizziness or fainting, fever, weight gain, palpitations, or irregular heartbeat. Fever may be a symptom of a concomitant infective or bacterial endocarditis.[58]

The evaluation of patients with suspected valvular disease revolves around confirming the diagnosis, quantifying the extent of the valvular abnormality, and assessing its consequences. Clinical evaluation should include a thorough history of current and past symptoms, especially those related to heart failure, as well as a meticulous physical examination and auscultation of the heart. Transthoracic echocardiography should be performed in all patients with suspected valvular disease. The European Association of Cardiovascular Imaging and the American Society of Echocardiography have established parameters to determine the extent of valvular disease through echocardiography.[59–61]

CMR is valuable in assessing the severity of valvular lesions, particularly in cases of valvular regurgitation. CMR can evaluate ventricular volumes and systolic function, which has implications for the precise management of associated comorbid conditions. Additionally, CMR can reliably detect concomitant abnormalities of the ascending aorta and exhibits high sensitivity in identifying the presence of myocardial fibrosis.[59]

The presence of NBTE should prompt an evaluation for associated infectious organisms, including blood cultures, as a significant number of these thrombotic valvular lesions can become secondarily infected, leading to bacteremia.[53]

There are no specific immunosuppressive therapies recommended for patients with valvular disorders and underlying autoimmune conditions. However, patients with SLE and APS who are diagnosed with NBTE should be placed on anticoagulation therapy to reduce the risk of embolic events.[53] The presence of concomitant infective endocarditis should prompt the use of intravenous antibiotics. Patients with SLE-associated NBTE should be monitored closely during anticoagulation therapy, as they are at a higher risk of developing thromboembolic events during this period. Scheduled echocardiography every 3–6 months is recommended to monitor the progression and resolution of these lesions.[62] Patients with progressive valvular disease leading to worsening dysfunction and symptoms should be evaluated by interventional cardiology for interventions geared toward preserving valve function. Surgical options for valvular repair or replacement by cardiothoracic surgery may also be considered in select patients where indicated.[59]

REFERENCES

1. Manolis AS, Tzioufas AG. Cardio-rheumatology: cardiovascular complications in systemic autoimmune rheumatic diseases/is inflammation the common link and target? Curr Vasc Pharmacol. 2020;18(5):425–430.
2. Lee KS, et al. Cardiovascular involvement in systemic rheumatic diseases: an integrated view for the treating physicians. Autoimmun Rev. 2018;17(3):201–214.
3. Chiabrando JG, et al. Management of acute and recurrent pericarditis: JACC state-of-the-art review. J Am Coll Cardiol. 2020;75(1):76–92.
4. Troughton RW, et al. Pericarditis. Lancet. 2004;363(9410):717–727.
5. Hinds SW, et al. Diagnosis of pericardial abnormalities by 2D-echo: a pathology-echocardiography correlation in 85 patients. Am Heart J. 1992;123(1):143–150.
6. Alraies MC, et al. Usefulness of cardiac magnetic resonance-guided management in patients with recurrent pericarditis. Am J Cardiol. 2015;115(4):542–547.
7. Adler Y, et al. 2015 ESC guidelines for the diagnosis and management of pericardial diseases: the task force for the diagnosis and management of pericardial diseases of the European Society of Cardiology (ESC) endorsed by: the European Association for Cardio-Thoracic Surgery (EACTS). Eur Heart J. 2015;36(42):2921–2964.
8. Permanyer-Miralda G. Acute pericardial disease: approach to the aetiologic diagnosis. Heart. 2004;90(3):252–254.
9. Imazio M, et al. Colchicine as first-choice therapy for recurrent pericarditis: results of the CORE (COlchicine for REcurrent pericarditis) trial. Arch Intern Med. 2005;165(17):1987–1991.
10. Imazio M, et al. A randomized trial of colchicine for acute pericarditis. N Engl J Med. 2013;369(16):1522–1528.
11. Lotrionte M, et al. International collaborative systematic review of controlled clinical trials on pharmacologic treatments for acute pericarditis and its recurrences. Am Heart J. 2010;160(4):662–670.
12. Brucato A, et al. Effect of anakinra on recurrent pericarditis among patients with colchicine resistance and corticosteroid dependence: the AIRTRIP randomized clinical trial. JAMA. 2016;316(18):1906–1912.
13. Wohlford GF, et al. Acute effects of interleukin-1 blockade using anakinra in patients with acute pericarditis. J Cardiovasc Pharmacol. 2020;76(1):50–52.
14. Kedor C, et al. Canakinumab for treatment of adult-onset Still's disease to achieve reduction of arthritic manifestation (CONSIDER): phase II, randomised, double-blind, placebo-controlled, multicentre, investigator-initiated trial. Ann Rheum Dis. 2020;79(8):1090–1097.
15. Taylor T, et al. Causes of death among individuals with systemic lupus erythematosus by race and ethnicity: a population-based study. Arthritis Care Res. 2023;75(1):61–68.
16. Schoenfeld SR, et al. The epidemiology of atherosclerotic cardiovascular disease among patients with SLE: a systematic review. Semin Arthritis Rheum. 2013;43(1):77–95.
17. Manzi S, Wasko MC. Inflammation-mediated rheumatic diseases and atherosclerosis. Ann Rheum Dis. 2000;59(5):321–325.
18. Katayama Y, et al. Risk factors for cardiovascular diseases in patients with systemic lupus erythematosus: an umbrella review. Clin Rheumatol. 2023;42(11):2931–2941.

19. Maradit-Kremers H, et al. Increased unrecognized coronary heart disease and sudden deaths in rheumatoid arthritis: a population-based cohort study. Arthritis Rheum. 2005;52(2):402–411.

20. Drosos GC, et al. EULAR recommendations for cardiovascular risk management in rheumatic and musculoskeletal diseases, including systemic lupus erythematosus and antiphospholipid syndrome. Ann Rheum Dis. 2022;81(6):768–779.

21. Petri MA, et al. Development of a systemic lupus erythematosus cardiovascular risk equation. Lupus Sci Med. 2019;6(1):e000346.

22. Melano-Carranza E, et al. Coronary artery disease in systemic lupus erythematosus: what do the facts say? Cureus. 2023;15(1):e33449.

23. Mendoza-Pinto C, et al. Asymptomatic coronary artery disease assessed by coronary computed tomography in patients with systemic lupus erythematosus: a systematic review and meta-analysis. Eur J Intern Med. 2022;100:102–109.

24. Birnie DH, et al. HRS expert consensus statement on the diagnosis and management of arrhythmias associated with cardiac sarcoidosis. Heart Rhythm. 2014;11(7):1305–1323.

25. Bissell LA, et al. Primary myocardial disease in scleroderma-a comprehensive review of the literature to inform the UK Systemic Sclerosis Study Group cardiac working group. Rheumatology. 2017;56(6):882–895.

26. Bissell LA, et al. Consensus best practice pathway of the UK Systemic Sclerosis Study group: management of cardiac disease in systemic sclerosis. Rheumatology. 2017;56(6):912–921.

27. Lindhardsen J, et al. Risk of atrial fibrillation and stroke in rheumatoid arthritis: Danish nationwide cohort study. BMJ. 2012 Mar 8;344:e1257.

28. Geraldino-Pardilla L, et al. ECG non-specific ST-T and QTc abnormalities in patients with systemic lupus erythematosus compared with rheumatoid arthritis. Lupus Sci Med. 2016;3(1):e000168.

29. Ammirati E, et al. Management of acute myocarditis and chronic inflammatory cardiomyopathy: an expert consensus document. Circ Heart Fail. 2020;13(11):e007405.

30. Witberg G, et al. Myocarditis after Covid-19 vaccination in a large health care organization. N Engl J Med. 2021;385(23):2132–2139.

31. Patone M, et al. Risk of myocarditis after sequential doses of COVID-19 vaccine and SARS-CoV-2 infection by age and sex. Circulation. 2022;146(10):743–754.

32. du Toit R, et al. Lupus myocarditis: review of current diagnostic modalities and their application in clinical practice. Rheumatology. 2023;62(2):523–534.

33. Kikuchi N, et al. Acute myocarditis complicating systemic lupus erythematosus: detection and evolution of transmural spiral late gadolinium enhancement on cardiac magnetic resonance imaging. Circ Cardiovasc Imaging. 2021 Feb;14(2):e011319.

34. Guglin M, et al. The spectrum of lupus myocarditis: from asymptomatic forms to cardiogenic shock. Heart Fail Rev. 2021;26(3):553–560.

35. Bruestle K, et al. Autoimmunity in acute myocarditis: how immunopathogenesis steers new directions for diagnosis and treatment. Curr Cardiol Rep. 2020;22(5):28.

36. Ammirati E, Moslehi JJ. Diagnosis and treatment of acute myocarditis: a review. JAMA. 2023;329(13): 1098–1113.

37. Caforio AL, et al. Current state of knowledge on aetiology, diagnosis, management, and therapy of myocarditis: a position statement of the European Society of Cardiology Working Group on Myocardial and Pericardial Diseases. Eur Heart J. 2013 Sep;34(33):2636–2648.

38. Bracamonte-Baran W, Čiháková D. Cardiac autoimmunity: myocarditis. Adv Exp Med Biol. 2017;1003:187–221.

39. Younis A, et al. Epidemiology characteristics and outcome of patients with clinically diagnosed acute myocarditis. Am J Med. 2020 Apr;133(4):492–499.

40. Ammirati E, et al. Clinical presentation and outcome in a contemporary cohort of patients with acute myocarditis: multicenter lombardy registry. Circulation. 2018;138(11):1088–1099.

41. Bennett MK, et al. Evaluation of the role of endomyocardial biopsy in 851 patients with unexplained heart failure from 2000-2009. Circ Heart Fail. 2013;6(4):676–684.

42. Agrawal T, et al. Diagnosis of cardiac sarcoidosis: a primer for non-imagers. Heart Fail Rev. 2022 Jul;27(4):1223–1233.

43. Mavrogeni S, et al. Silent myocarditis in systemic sclerosis detected by cardiovascular magnetic resonance using Lake Louise criteria. BMC Cardiovasc Disord. 2017;17(1):187.

44. Friedrich MG, et al. Cardiovascular magnetic resonance in myocarditis: a JACC White Paper. J Am Coll Cardiol. 2009;53(17):1475–1487.

45. Birnie DH, et al. Cardiac sarcoidosis. J Am Coll Cardiol. 2016;68(4):411–421.

46. Berg J, et al. Non-steroidal anti-inflammatory drug use in acute myopericarditis: 12-month clinical follow-up. Open Heart. 2019 Apr 23;6(1):e000990.

47. Ammirati E, et al. Immunomodulating therapies in acute myocarditis and recurrent/acute pericarditis. Front Med. 2022;9:838564.

48. McNamara DM, et al. Intravenous immune globulin in the therapy of myocarditis and acute cardiomyopathy. Circulation. 1997 Jun 3;95(11):2476–2478.

49. Kishimoto C, et al. Therapy with immunoglobulin in patients with acute myocarditis and cardiomyopathy: analysis of leukocyte balance. Heart Vessels. 2014;29(3):336–342.

50. Zuily S, et al. Increased risk for heart valve disease associated with antiphospholipid antibodies in patients with systemic lupus erythematosus: meta-analysis of echocardiographic studies. Circulation. 2011 Jul 12;124(2):215–224.

51. Hussain K, et al. A meta-analysis and systematic review of valvular heart disease in systemic lupus erythematosus and its association with antiphospholipid antibodies. J Clin Rheumatol. 2021;27(8):e525–e532.

52. Farhat H, et al. Increased risk of cardiovascular diseases in rheumatoid arthritis: a systematic review. Cureus. 2022;14(12):e32308.

53. Katsouli A, Massad MG. Current issues in the diagnosis and management of blood culture-negative infective and non-infective endocarditis. Ann Thorac Surg. 2013;95(4):1467–1474.

54. Kitas G, Banks MJ, Bacon PA. Cardiac involvement in rheumatoid disease. Clin Med. 2001;1(1):18–21.

55. Maksimowicz-McKinnon K, Mandell BF. Understanding valvular heart disease in patients with systemic autoimmune diseases. Cleve Clin J Med. 2004;71(11):881–885.

56. Kurmann RD, et al. Increased risk of valvular heart disease in systemic sclerosis: an underrecognized cardiac complication. J Rheumatol. 2021;48(7):1047–1052.

57. Pan SY, et al. Cardiac damage in autoimmune diseases: target organ involvement that cannot be ignored. Front Immunol. 2022;13:1056400.

58. Otto CM, Bonow RO. "Valvular heart disease: A companion to Braunwald's heart disease." In Valvular Heart Disease: A Companion to Braunwald's Heart Disease Expert Consult-Online and Print 2009 (pp. 1–452). Elsevier.

59. Vahanian A, et al. 2021 ESC/EACTS guidelines for the management of valvular heart disease. Eur Heart J. 2022 Feb 12;43(7):561–632.

60. Baumgartner H, et al. Recommendations on the echocardiographic assessment of aortic valve stenosis: a focused update from the European Association of Cardiovascular Imaging and the American Society of Echocardiography. Eur Heart J Cardiovasc Imaging. 2017;18(3):254–275.

61. Lancellotti P, et al. Recommendations for the echocardiographic assessment of native valvular regurgitation: an executive summary from the European Association of Cardiovascular Imaging. Eur Heart J Cardiovasc Imaging. 2013 Jul;14(7):611–44.

62. Tayem MG, et al. A review of cardiac manifestations in patients with systemic lupus erythematosus and antiphospholipid syndrome with focus on endocarditis. Cureus. 2022;14(1):e21698.

2

Fundamental principles of cardiac imaging and other diagnostic testing in patients with rheumatic disease

GIZEM BILGILI AND JANET WEI

INTRODUCTION

Given the various cardiac manifestations of autoimmune rheumatic diseases, diagnostic tools are essential to the investigation and management of these patients with cardiac symptoms.[1] Testing strategies depend on the suspicion for ischemic heart disease, myocarditis, arrhythmias, valve dysfunction, pulmonary hypertension, heart failure, and vascular inflammation (Table 2.1).[2–4] This chapter will review fundamental principles of cardiac imaging and other diagnostic testing in patients with rheumatic disease.

Blood biomarkers

TROPONIN

Cardiac troponin is a specific marker for myocardial cell damage and necrosis and can be elevated in settings of myocardial ischemia and injury, such as acute myocardial infarction (MI) and myocarditis. The American College of Cardiology (ACC)/American Heart Association (AHA) guidelines recommend measuring cardiac troponin in the evaluation and diagnosis of acute chest pain as a class 1 recommendation, with high-sensitivity cardiac troponin as the preferred biomarker.[5] The 99th percentile upper reference limits are recommended as the threshold for myocardial injury or infarction, and high-sensitivity assays have been shown to shorten the length of stay in the emergency department for ruling out MI.[6] Since the majority of patients diagnosed with autoimmune rheumatic diseases are women,[7] it is important to note that women have lower 99th percentiles than men, and sex-specific thresholds improve the underdiagnosis of women with acute MI.[6]

Among patients with systemic lupus erythematosus (SLE), rheumatoid arthritis (RA), and systemic sclerosis (SSc) without pre-existing cardiovascular disease, high-sensitivity cardiac troponin is elevated compared to healthy controls, independent of cardiovascular risk factors.[8–10] High-sensitivity cardiac troponin is related to disease activity and inflammatory markers, supporting the link between myocardial injury and inflammation.[10]

NATRIURETIC PEPTIDE

Natriuretic peptides, B-type natriuretic peptide (BNP) and N-terminal proBNP (NT-proBNP), are released from cardiac myocytes in ventricles in response to volume or pressure overload, and thus, they are used to diagnose and monitor heart failure.[11] BNP and NT-proBNP levels may be influenced by age, race, sex, body mass index,

DOI: 10.1201/9781003386711-2

Table 2.1 Comparison of cardiovascular imaging approaches for autoimmune rheumatic diseases[4]

CVD manifestation	ECHO	SPECT	PET	CT	CMR
Myocardial ischemia	++	+++	++++	−	++++
Coronary anatomy	−	−	+	+++	++[a]
Pericarditis[b]	+++	−	−	++	++++
Myocarditis	+/−	−	+/−	−	++++
Heart failure	+++	++	++	++	++++
Pulmonary hypertension	++++	−	−	−	+++
Valvular disease	++++	−	−	−	+++
Vascular inflammation	+/−	−	+++	++	+++

Note: CVD, cardiovascular disease; ECHO, echocardiography; SPECT, single-photon emission computed tomography; PET, positron emission tomography; CT, computed tomography; CMR, cardiovascular magnetic resonance.

[a] Pediatric patients.
[b] Particularly, pericarditis without effusion can be detected by CMR by positive LGE of the pericardium.

and renal function. While circulating levels of natriuretic peptides are generally higher in those with heart failure with reduced ejection fraction (HFrEF) than heart failure with preserved ejection (HFpEF), elevated levels reflect heart failure disease severity and associated with worse clinical outcomes and mortality.[11]

Inflammation has been associated with natriuretic peptide release, hypothesized due to myocardial wall strain, cardiac neurohormonal derangement, and myocardial ischemia.[12,13] NT-proBNP has been demonstrated to be elevated in RA and SLE patients[10,14] and appears to be an early marker of subclinical cardiovascular involvement in various autoimmune rheumatic diseases.[15,16] The presence of high natriuretic peptide levels in SSc patients should raise concern for biventricular cardiac dysfunction and fibrosis, as well as SSc-related pulmonary arterial hypertension (PAH).[13,17]

Evaluation of arrhythmias

ELECTROCARDIOGRAPHY (ECG)

ECG is an inexpensive, easily reproducible diagnostic and prognostic tool, providing information on heart rate, rhythm, chamber size and morphology, ischemia, and infarction. ST-T changes and QT prolongation are associated with increased mortality risk.[18]

In autoimmune rheumatic diseases, the most common ECG abnormalities are sinus tachycardia, nonspecific ST segment changes, QT prolongation, and tachyarrhythmia with a predominance of atrial fibrillation.[19–21] QT prolongation has previously been associated with inflammatory marker levels in patients with RA.[22] Acquired long QT syndrome can occur in the setting of anti-Ro/SSA-positive connective tissue disease, while anti-Ro/SSA antibodies can also induce sinoatrial node dysfunction and atrial-ventricular block in patients and in the offspring of anti-Ro/SSA-positive mothers.[23] Autoimmune diseases are significantly associated with the risk of atrial fibrillation, particularly in women.[24]

AMBULATORY ELECTROCARDIOGRAPHIC (ECG) MONITORING

Ambulatory monitoring is often prescribed for the evaluation of palpitations or syncope/presyncope, as it can assess the health of the cardiac conduction system and detect supraventricular and ventricular arrhythmias.[19] Ambulatory ECG monitoring can range from 24 to 48 hours (Holter monitoring) or up to 30 days (event monitoring). Wearable adhesive "patch" ECG monitors typically record 1- or 2-lead electrogram, can be worn continuously for up to 14 days, and allow patients to press a button to mark symptomatic episodes.[25] Implantable loop recorders may help record cardiac electrical activity for up to 3 years and may be prescribed in patients with recurrent palpitations, syncope of unclear etiology, or when shorter monitoring has been unrevealing. Among SS patients, ambulatory ECG monitors have detected a high prevalence of supraventricular and ventricular ectopy or arrhythmias, and those with arrhythmias and poor prognosis tend to be those with concomitant skeletal and cardiac muscle involvement.[26] Screening monitors to detect cardiac conduction and repolarization abnormalities in patients with SLE and anti-Ro/SSA positivity are not recommended.[27]

Evaluation of structural heart disease (pericardial, valvular, and myocardial) and pulmonary hypertension

ECHOCARDIOGRAPHY

Transthoracic echocardiography (TTE) is a reliable, easily accessible, and low-cost imaging technique that can diagnose a variety of cardiac abnormalities and may also be used repeatedly to track disease progression and evaluate response to treatment.[28]

Pericardial effusion, inflammation, and thickening are the most common cardiac manifestations in patients with RA, SLE, and SSc.[28] In healthy individuals, there is approximately 50 mL plasma filtrate between the visceral and parietal pericardial layers which can be seen only during systole.[29] Pericardial effusion is diagnosed when fluid accumulates between these two layers, and the separation of these layers is visible during the entire cardiac cycle.[28,29] In the setting of rapid or large pericardial effusion accumulation, cardiac tamponade can occur, which can cause hemodynamic compromise (Figure 2.1). Echocardiographic findings of cardiac tamponade include right ventricular early diastolic collapse, right atrial late diastolic collapse, absence of inspiratory collapse of the inferior vena cava, and the swinging of the entire heart.[28,29] Constrictive pericarditis may develop in patients with chronic or recurrent pericarditis, leading to thickened and rigid pericardium with dissociation of intrathoracic and intracardiac pressures. Tissue Doppler echocardiography can be useful to see diastolic and pulmonary blood flow changes on cardiac tamponade and constrictive pericarditis.[28]

Valvular diseases associated with SLE include valvular thickening, vegetations, and insufficiency. Libman–Sacks endocarditis is characterized by nonbacterial vegetations <10 mm and occurs in patients with antiphospholipid syndrome. These verrucous lesions can be various shapes with irregular borders on different densities, and they usually position aortic or mitral leaflets.[28,30] Transesophageal echocardiography (TEE) is more sensitive than TTE for evaluating structural and functional abnormalities of the cardiac valves. The valves can be further visualized with 3D TEE, which can guide surgical and interventional procedures.

Myocardial disease contributing to congestive heart failure can occur in autoimmune rheumatic diseases, including SS which is characterized by abnormal collagen accumulation and fibrosis.

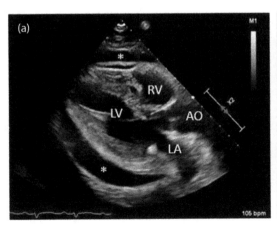 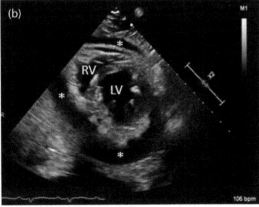

Figure 2.1 **Pericardial effusion diagnosis by echocardiography.** Transthoracic echocardiogram demonstrating a moderate circumferential pericardial effusion (*) in the parasternal long-axis (A) and short-axis (B) views, in an elderly woman with polymyalgia rheumatica and new-onset shortness of breath. AO, aorta; LA, left atrium; LV, left ventricle; RV, right ventricle.

Echocardiographic measures of myocardial disease and heart failure include increased chamber sizes, impaired systolic and diastolic function, and signs of elevated filling pressures.[31,32] Tissue Doppler echocardiography can be used to measure systolic and diastolic myocardial flow velocity.[31]

Speckle tracking echocardiography (STE) assesses myocardial strain by measuring the deformation or lengthening/shortening of myocardial tissue.[33] STE tracks the movement of echogenic speckles in the left ventricular wall to measure strain as a percentage change in the dimension of a speckle from one time point to another.[34] STE is particularly advantageous over tissue Doppler echocardiography in the early stages of rheumatic diseases as it enables investigation of the disposition of myocardial segments and myocardial deformation in three dimensions (radial, circumferential, and longitudinal).[31,35] For patients with RA, STE can detect subclinical myocardial dysfunction,[34,35] possibly related to prolonged inflammation and excessive cytokine-induced fibroblast activity leading to defective endothelial and microcirculatory function, resulting in diminished left ventricular longitudinal and circumferential strain.[34] In studies of RA patients treated with TNF and interleukin inhibitors, improvements in global longitudinal strain have been observed, although large clinical trials are needed.[35] In early Behçet's disease, microvascular inflammation and endomyocardial fibrosis due to exaggerated fibroblast activation may result in impaired longitudinal strain despite normal traditional systolic parameters and preserved circumferential strain.[36] In SLE, reductions in left ventricular longitudinal, radial, and circumferential strains represent early signs of cardiac damage in the absence of left ventricular ejection fraction reduction.[37] In acute lupus myocarditis, midmyocardial and epicardial function stays relatively unaffected, and circumferential strain is modified to compensate left ventricular systolic dysfunction.[38] Finally, both impaired left ventricular strain and right ventricular strain can be seen in SS compared to healthy subjects, reflecting cardiac and pulmonary manifestations of SS.[39]

Myocardial contrast echocardiography (MCE) is a method for assessing the myocardial microcirculation, in which intravenous infusion of gas-filled microbubbles allows the detection of region of MI and assessment of the success of reperfusion and extent of viable myocardium.[40] MCE for the evaluation of coronary microvascular dysfunction is currently a research tool and has not been studied extensively in autoimmune rheumatic disease settings.

CARDIAC MAGNETIC RESONANCE IMAGING (MRI)

Cardiac MRI is considered the gold standard noninvasive imaging modality for determining structural and functional cardiovascular complications of autoimmune rheumatologic diseases, providing accurate and reproducible operator-independent images.[3,4,41] Cardiac MRI images are based on signals arising from hydrogen nuclei, which are excited by a radiofrequency wave pulse sequence. The longitudinal and transverse relaxation processes of the net proton vector are termed T1 and T2 relaxation. T1-weighted spin echo sequences are typically used for anatomical assessment, gradient-echo (bright-blood steady-state-free precession) cine sequences in short axis and long-axis planes to evaluate cardiac function and chamber volumes. T2-weighted spin echo sequences provide images about acute, predominantly tissue edema. CMR is frequently used in the evaluation of heart failure and myocarditis in patients with autoimmune rheumatic diseases.[3,33,41]

Gadolinium-contrast enhanced inversion-recovery gradient-echo sequences with appropriate nulling of normal myocardium are used to assess for late gadolinium enhancement (LGE), which appears as bright white tissue representative of replacement myocardial fibrosis.[3] Specific patterns of LGE represent MI (subendocardial or transmural in a vascular distribution), myocarditis (midwall or epicardial LGE, often patchy), or other cardiomyopathies.

T1 mapping and T2 mapping enable rapid tissue characterization in patients with autoimmune rheumatic disease.[31,32] Among patients with SLE, RA, spondyloarthropathy, and SS, inflammatory cardiomyopathy is a serious complication resulting from repetitive myocardial injury.[42] T1 and T2 mapping, as well as the measurement of extracellular volume, reflect diffuse myocardial fibrosis, edema, and inflammation.[42] In SLE patients with suspected lupus myocarditis, T1 and T2 relaxation times are elevated, but these CMR measures may not correlate with SLE disease activity and inflammatory or cardiac biomarkers. Nevertheless, T1 and T2 mapping may help detect subclinical myocardial injury and overt myocarditis.[33] Diagnosis of myocarditis using the Lake Louise Criteria requires the presence of acute edema/inflammation on T2 imaging as well as evidence of fibrosis or scar by T1 or LGE imaging.[43] In SS patients with inflammatory cardiomyopathy, a CMR score combining T2 and LGE data can help predict risk of ventricular arrhythmias.[41,44]

Cardiac MRI can also reveal pericardial diseases that are frequent cardiac manifestations of autoimmune rheumatic diseases.[4] Pericardial effusions can be quantified, and native T1 mapping can help distinguish between transudative and exudative pericardial effusions.[45] The presence of pericardial LGE represents pericardial inflammation consistent with pericarditis and may guide anti-inflammatory treatment.[46]

CARDIAC COMPUTED TOMOGRAPHY (CT)

Cardiac CT is widely available, non-invasive imaging technique that uses iodine-based contrast to visualize cardiac structure and function.[3,4,32] Cardiac CT may be reasonable for determining the presence and degree of pericardial thickening in patients with acute chest pain and suspected acute pericarditis (ACC/AHA class 2b).[5]

Evaluation of coronary artery disease and dysfunction

STRESS TESTING

For low-risk patients with autoimmune disease, no known coronary artery disease (CAD), and interpretable ECG, exercise treadmill testing without imaging is reasonable for excluding myocardial ischemia and determining functional capacity (ACC/AHA class 2a recommendation).[5] Functional stress testing with imaging (echocardiography, nuclear, or MRI) is recommended as a class 1 indication for the evaluation of stable chest pain in intermediate- or high-risk patients to assess the presence of hemodynamically significant coronary stenosis.[5]

Stress echocardiography with exercise or pharmacological provocation is able to detect hemodynamic changes in cardiac and pulmonary vascular system.[47,48] For those who are unable to exercise, pharmacological stress echocardiography can be conducted with dobutamine, dipyridamole, or adenosine infusions.[3] Stress echocardiography allows the evaluation of myocardial and valvular function and pulmonary hypertension during stress. For diagnosis of pulmonary hypertension, stress echocardiography is more advantageous than resting echocardiography in patients with SS, SLE, and mixed connective tissue disease as the diagnosis may help lead to early initiation of treatment.[2,47,48] Doppler echocardiography of the left anterior descending artery during pharmacologic stress can also be useful for diagnosing coronary microvascular dysfunction (ACC/AHA class 2b).[5]

Nuclear perfusion imaging such as single-photon emission computed tomography (SPECT) is frequently used in clinical cardiology for the prediction of obstructive CAD, but it has some disadvantages which include using radioactive tracers, low spatial resolution, and high cost.[31,32] Similar to SPECT, stress cardiac positron emission tomography (PET) has high sensitivity and specificity for detecting obstructive CAD, but cardiac PET is associated with lower radiation and better diagnostic performance when compared with SPECT.[32] Rest and vasodilator stress PET can quantify myocardial blood flow for measurement of myocardial flow reserve in autoimmune patients with suspected coronary microvascular dysfunction (ACC/AHA class 2a) (Figure 2.2).[49]

Stress cardiac MRI is an emerging diagnostic and prognostic tool for evaluating myocardial ischemia and may have distinct advantages in autoimmune rheumatic disease patients due to concomitant assessment of myocardial and pericardial structure, function, inflammation, and fibrosis. Patients without CMR perfusion defects or LGE are at low risk for cardiac events and coronary revascularization.[50] Semi-quantitative measurement of myocardial perfusion reserve index (MPRI) predicts coronary microvascular dysfunction in patients with angina and no obstructive CAD,[51] predicts worse prognosis if impaired,[52] and is often impaired in patients with SLE and persistent chest pain.[53,54] Among women with coronary microvascular dysfunction, those with history of autoimmune rheumatic disease have lower MPRI than those without autoimmune rheumatic disease, suggesting worse microvascular function.[55] Semi-quantitative or fully quantitative measurement of coronary microvascular dysfunction is reasonable for patients with persistent stable chest pain and no obstructive CAD (ACC/AHA class 2a).[5]

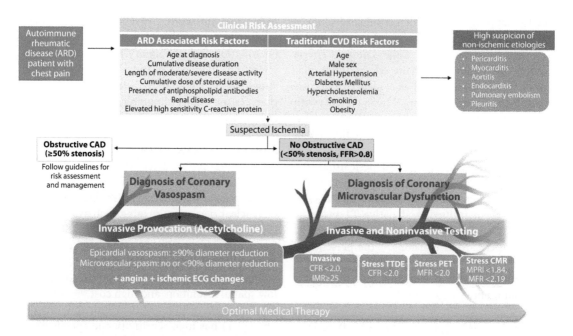

Figure 2.2 Clinical algorithm for risk assessment of autoimmune rheumatic disease (ARD) patients with chest pain and diagnosis of coronary microvascular dysfunction and vasospasm. Non-invasive testing and invasive testing allow assessment of coronary microvascular dysfunction, while invasive acetylcholine provocation testing can additionally assess coronary vasospasm. CAD, coronary artery disease; CFR, coronary flow reserve; CMR, cardiac magnetic resonance imaging; CVD, cardiovascular disease; ECG, electrocardiogram; FFR, fractional flow reserve; IMR, index of microcirculatory restriction; MFR, myocardial flow reserve; MPRI, myocardial perfusion reserve index; PET, positron emission tomography; and TTDE, transthoracic Doppler echocardiography. (Adapted with permission Ref. [49].)

CORONARY CT ANGIOGRAPHY

Cardiac CT can provide diagnostic and prognostic coronary evaluation with or without contrast. Coronary artery calcium (CAC) can be visualized and quantified using non-contrast cardiac CT, and it is a useful diagnostic and prognostic test for coronary atherosclerosis, with higher scores indicating increased cardiac risk. CAC significantly improves risk prediction beyond traditional risk factors and is recommended to improve cardiovascular risk prediction for borderline-to-intermediate risk patients.[56] CAC studies suggest that CAC scores are higher in patients with autoimmune rheumatic diseases compared to controls, possibly due to chronic inflammation.[57] For low-risk patients with stable chest pain and no known CAD, CAC may be considered for excluding calcified plaque and identifying patients with low likelihood of obstructive CAD (ACC/AHA class 2a).[5] For intermediate- or high-risk patients with stable chest pain, coronary CT angiography is recommended to identify obstructive CAD (≥50% stenosis) (ACC/AHA class 1)[5] and can quantify plaque burden and high-risk plaque features.[58,59] For intermediate stenosis, functional flow reserve by CT ($FFR_{CT}\leq0.8$) indicates hemodynamically significant stenosis that may benefit from revascularization.[60]

INVASIVE CORONARY ANGIOGRAPHY, INTRACORONARY IMAGING, AND CORONARY FUNCTION TESTING

Invasive coronary angiography is the gold standard for diagnosis of obstructive CAD or other flow limiting lesions such as spontaneous coronary artery dissection (SCAD). Invasive coronary angiography is recommended for the evaluation of patients with acute chest pain and high-risk CAD, frequent angina, or evidence of moderate-to-severe ischemia on stress testing (ACC/AHA class 1).[5]

Although SCAD has been reported in the setting of autoimmune rheumatic diseases, a recent case-control study suggests that autoimmune diseases are not associated with SCAD.[61] Intracoronary imaging with intravascular ultrasound or optical coherence tomography, along with cardiac MRI, may be helpful for determining mechanism of MI in the setting of no obstructive coronary arteries.[62] For patients with signs and symptoms of ischemia and no obstructive CAD, invasive coronary function testing offers comprehensive evaluation for the diagnosis of coronary microvascular dysfunction and coronary vasospasm and enhancement of risk stratification (ACC/AHA class 2a).[5,63,64]

Evaluation of aortic disease

Aortitis is associated with giant cell arthritis, Takayasu arteritis, granulomatosis with polyangiitis, polyarteritis nodosa, SLE, RA, and Behçet's disease.[65] To diagnosing autoimmune aortic disease, different methods might be useful such as tissue biopsy, echocardiography, FDG PET, and CT angiography. Invasiveness and patchy/uneven distribution of disease make tissue biopsy less preferable than imaging modalities.[32,66]

Ultrasound, including echocardiography, can identify aortitis as thickening of the aortic wall with surrounding edema.[66,67] Ultrasound can also diagnose complications of aortitis: Aortic aneurysm, dissection, hematoma, and penetrating ulcer.[66] In Takayasu arteritis, a homogenous, circumferential wall thickening accompanied by stenosis is described as the "macaroni sign" and is a rare but pathognomonic finding.[68] Tissue Doppler imaging provides additional information of arterial flow in patients with weak or absent pulses, claudication, and digit ulcerations.[66]

Fluorodeoxyglucose (FDG)-PET imaging is suitable for assessing inflammation intramural aortic wall and periaortic areas that utilized by monocytes. In regions of inflammation, excess 18F-FDG uptake may be visualized and may guide tissue biopsy and understanding of disease severity and response to treatment. FDG PET can be used in patients with chronic kidney impairment and metal implants who are not eligible for MRI.[20] In Takayasu arteritis, FDG PET can show disease involvement in extracranial arteries, but exaggerated FDG uptake can also be observed in atherosclerosis, vascular fibrosis, and remodeling in the absence of acute inflammation.

For subjects without significant renal impairment, CT angiography is an important diagnostic tool for diagnosing large vessel vasculitis.[4] CTA demonstrates thickening of aortic wall, periaortic inflammation, and wall edema in setting of rheumatologic aortic diseases especially giant cell arthritis.[65] In Takayasu arthritis, mural thickening can be seen as double ring sign in large vessels, representing inflamed media and adventitia.[66] In Behçet's disease, CT angiography is useful to detect systemic, aortic, and pulmonary aneurysms; aortitis is a rare but severe complication, sometimes involving the aortic root and leading to aortic regurgitation.[69]

Magnetic resonance angiography can detect large vessel aneurysms and wall edema in patients with giant cell arthritis.[66] In Takayasu arteritis, MRA with LGE can evaluate severity of stenosis as well as distinguish between active and stable arteritis.[70]

CONCLUSION

Cardiac imaging and other diagnostic testing are essential in the evaluation of cardiac disease in patients with autoimmune rheumatic disease. Cardiac testing allows the identification of subclinical abnormalities, frank disease, and prognosis. Data is limited regarding how the diagnostic modalities should be used to guide treatment to improve outcomes in patients with autoimmune rheumatic diseases.

REFERENCES

1. Sen G, Gordon P, Sado DM. Cardiac manifestations of rheumatological disease: a synopsis for the cardiologist. Heart. 2021;107(14):1173–1181.
2. Makavos G, Varoudi M, Papangelopoulou K, Kapniari E, Plotas P, Ikonomidis I, et al. Echocardiography in autoimmune rheumatic diseases for diagnosis and prognosis of cardiovascular complications. Medicina. 2020;56(9):445.
3. Atzeni F, Corda M, Gianturco L, Porcu M, Sarzi-Puttini P, Turiel M. Cardiovascular imaging techniques in systemic rheumatic diseases. Front Med. 2018;5:26.

4. Mavrogeni S, Pepe A, Nijveldt R, Ntusi N, Sierra-Galan LM, Bratis K, et al. Cardiovascular magnetic resonance in autoimmune rheumatic diseases: a clinical consensus document by the European Association of Cardiovascular Imaging. Eur Heart J Cardiovasc Imaging. 2022;23(9):e308–e322.

5. Gulati M, Levy PD, Mukherjee D, Amsterdam E, Bhatt DL, Birtcher KK, et al. 2021 AHA/ACC/ASE/Chest/SAEM/SCCT/SCMR guideline for the evaluation and diagnosis of chest pain: a report of the American College of Cardiology/American Heart Association Joint Committee on Clinical Practice Guidelines. J Am Coll Cardiol. 2021;78(22):e187–e285.

6. Sandoval Y, Apple FS, Mahler SA, Body R, Collinson PO, Jaffe AS, et al. High-sensitivity cardiac troponin and the 2021 AHA/ACC/ASE/CHEST/SAEM/SCCT/SCMR guidelines for the evaluation and diagnosis of acute chest pain. Circulation. 2022;146(7):569–581.

7. Fairweather D, Rose NR. Women and autoimmune diseases. Emerg Infect Dis. 2004;10(11):2005–2011.

8. Divard G, Abbas R, Chenevier-Gobeaux C, Chanson N, Escoubet B, Chauveheid MP, et al. High-sensitivity cardiac troponin T is a biomarker for atherosclerosis in systemic lupus erythematous patients: a cross-sectional controlled study. Arthritis Res Ther. 2017;19(1):132.

9. Avouac J, Meune C, Chenevier-Gobeaux C, Borderie D, Lefevre G, Kahan A, et al. Cardiac biomarkers in systemic sclerosis: contribution of high-sensitivity cardiac troponin in addition to N-terminal pro-brain natriuretic peptide. Arthritis Care Res. 2015;67(7):1022–1030.

10. Avouac J, Meune C, Chenevier-Gobeaux C, Dieude P, Borderie D, Lefevre G, et al. Inflammation and disease activity are associated with high circulating cardiac markers in rheumatoid arthritis independently of traditional cardiovascular risk factors. J Rheumatol. 2014;41(2):248–255.

11. Chow SL, Maisel AS, Anand I, Bozkurt B, de Boer RA, Felker GM, et al. Role of biomarkers for the prevention, assessment, and management of heart failure: a scientific statement from the American Heart Association. Circulation. 2017;135(22):e1054–e1091.

12. Fish-Trotter H, Ferguson JF, Patel N, Arora P, Allen NB, Bachmann KN, et al. Inflammation and circulating natriuretic peptide levels. Circ Heart Fail. 2020;13(7):e006570.

13. Dimitroulas T, Giannakoulas G, Karvounis H, Garyfallos A, Settas L, Kitas G. B-type natriuretic peptide in rheumatic diseases: a cardiac biomarker or a sophisticated acute phase reactant? Autoimmun Rev. 2012;11(12):837–843.

14. Goldenberg D, Miller E, Perna M, Sattar N, Welsh P, Roman MJ, et al. Association of N-terminal pro-brain natriuretic peptide with cardiac disease, but not with vascular disease, in systemic lupus erythematosus. Arthritis Rheum. 2012;64(1):316–317.

15. Harney SM, Timperley J, Daly C, Harin A, James T, Brown MA, et al. Brain natriuretic peptide is a potentially useful screening tool for the detection of cardiovascular disease in patients with rheumatoid arthritis. Ann Rheum Dis. 2006;65(1):136.

16. Allanore Y, Wahbi K, Borderie D, Weber S, Kahan A, Meune C. N-terminal pro-brain natriuretic peptide in systemic sclerosis: a new cornerstone of cardiovascular assessment? Ann Rheum Dis. 2009;68(12):1885–1889.

17. Allanore Y, Borderie D, Avouac J, Zerkak D, Meune C, Hachulla E, et al. High N-terminal pro-brain natriuretic peptide levels and low diffusing capacity for carbon monoxide as independent predictors of the occurrence of precapillary pulmonary arterial hypertension in patients with systemic sclerosis. Arthritis Rheum. 2008;58(1):284–291.

18. Rautaharju PM, Surawicz B, Gettes LS, Bailey JJ, Childers R, Deal BJ, et al. AHA/ACCF/HRS recommendations for the standardization and interpretation of the electrocardiogram: part IV: the ST segment, T and U waves, and the QT interval: a scientific statement from The American Heart Association Electrocardiography and Arrhythmias

Committee, Council on Clinical Cardiology; The American College of Cardiology Foundation; and The Heart Rhythm Society: endorsed by The International Society for Computerized Electrocardiology. Circulation. 2009;119(10):e241–e250.

19. Lee KS, Kronbichler A, Eisenhut M, Lee KH, Shin JI. Cardiovascular involvement in systemic rheumatic diseases: an integrated view for the treating physicians. Autoimmun Rev. 2018;17(3):201–214.

20. Perel-Winkler A, Bokhari S, Perez-Recio T, Zartoshti A, Askanase A, Geraldino-Pardilla L. Myocarditis in systemic lupus erythematosus diagnosed by (18)F-fluorodeoxyglucose positron emission tomography. Lupus Sci Med. 2018;5(1):e000265.

21. Geraldino-Pardilla L, Gartshteyn Y, Pina P, Cerrone M, Giles JT, Zartoshti A, et al. ECG non-specific ST-T and QTc abnormalities in patients with systemic lupus erythematosus compared with rheumatoid arthritis. Lupus Sci Med. 2016;3(1):e000168.

22. Adlan AM, Panoulas VF, Smith JP, Fisher JP, Kitas GD. Association between corrected QT interval and inflammatory cytokines in rheumatoid arthritis. J Rheumatol. 2015;42(3):421–428.

23. Lazzerini PE, Capecchi PL, El-Sherif N, Laghi-Pasini F, Boutjdir M. Emerging arrhythmic risk of autoimmune and inflammatory cardiac channelopathies. J Am Heart Assoc. 2018;7(22):e010595.

24. Tilly MJ, Geurts S, Zhu F, Bos MM, Ikram MA, de Maat MPM, et al. Autoimmune diseases and new-onset atrial fibrillation: a UK Biobank study. Europace. 2023;25(3):804–811.

25. Steinberg JS, Varma N, Cygankiewicz I, Aziz P, Balsam P, Baranchuk A, et al. 2017 ISHNE-HRS expert consensus statement on ambulatory ECG and external cardiac monitoring/telemetry. Heart Rhythm. 2017;14(7):e55–e96.

26. Vacca A, Meune C, Gordon J, Chung L, Proudman S, Assassi S, et al. Cardiac arrhythmias and conduction defects in systemic sclerosis. Rheumatology (Oxford. 2014;53(7):1172–1177.

27. Villuendas R, Martinez-Morillo M, Junca G, Teniente-Serra A, Diez C, Heredia S, et al. Usefulness of cardiac screening in patients with systemic lupus erythematosus and anti-Ro/SSA antibodies. Lupus. 2021;30(10):1596–602.

28. Maksimovic R, Seferovic PM, Ristic AD, Vujisic-Tesic B, Simeunovic DS, Radovanovic G, et al. Cardiac imaging in rheumatic diseases. Rheumatology (Oxford). 2006;45(Suppl 4):iv26–31.

29. Goldar G, Garraud C, Sifuentes AA, Wassif H, Jain V, Klein AL. Autoimmune pericarditis: multimodality imaging. Curr Cardiol Rep. 2022;24(11):1633–1645.

30. Al Riyami H, Joshi N, Al Senaidi K, Al 'Abdul Salam N, Abdwani R. All endocarditis is not infective: Libman-Sacks endocarditis. Cureus. 2022;14(7):e26526.

31. Kumar K, Seetharam K, Poonam F, Gulati A, Sadiq A, Shetty V. The role of cardiac imaging in the evaluation of cardiac involvement in systemic diseases. Cureus. 2021;13(12):e20708.

32. Mavrogeni SI, Markousis-Mavrogenis G, Koutsogeorgopoulou L, Dimitroulas T, Vartela V, Rigopoulos A, et al. Pathophysiology and imaging of heart failure in women with autoimmune rheumatic diseases. Heart Fail Rev. 2019;24(4):489–498.

33. du Toit R, Karamchand S, Doubell AF, Reuter H, Herbst PG. Lupus myocarditis: review of current diagnostic modalities and their application in clinical practice. Rheumatology (Oxford). 2023;62(2):523–534.

34. Fine NM, Crowson CS, Lin G, Oh JK, Villarraga HR, Gabriel SE. Evaluation of myocardial function in patients with rheumatoid arthritis using strain imaging by speckle-tracking echocardiography. Ann Rheum Dis. 2014;73(10):1833–1839.

35. Thallapally VK, Bansal R, Thandra A, Gupta S, Aurit S, Pajjuru VS, et al. Detection of myocardial dysfunction using global longitudinal strain with speckle-tracking echocardiography in

patients with vs without rheumatoid arthritis: a systematic review and meta-analysis. J Echocardiogr. 2023;21(1):23–32.

36. Yagmur J, Sener S, Acikgoz N, Cansel M, Ermis N, Karincaoglu Y, et al. Subclinical left ventricular dysfunction in Behcet's disease assessed by two-dimensional speckle tracking echocardiography. Eur J Echocardiogr. 2011;12(7):536–541.

37. Di Minno MND, Forte F, Tufano A, Buonauro A, Rossi FW, De Paulis A, et al. Speckle tracking echocardiography in patients with systemic lupus erythematosus: a meta-analysis. Eur J Intern Med. 2020;73:16–22.

38. Du Toit R, Herbst PG, van Rensburg A, Snyman HW, Reuter H, Doubell AF. Speckle tracking echocardiography in acute lupus myocarditis: comparison to conventional echocardiography. Echo Res Pract. 2017;4(2):9–19.

39. Qiao W, Bi W, Wang X, Li Y, Ren W, Xiao Y. Cardiac involvement assessment in systemic sclerosis using speckle tracking echocardiography: a systematic review and meta-analysis. BMJ Open. 2023;13(2):e063364.

40. Lepper W, Belcik T, Wei K, Lindner JR, Sklenar J, Kaul S. Myocardial contrast echocardiography. Circulation. 2004;109(25):3132–3135.

41. Mavrogeni SI, Markousis-Mavrogenis G, Aggeli C, Tousoulis D, Kitas GD, Kolovou G, et al. Arrhythmogenic inflammatory cardiomyopathy in autoimmune rheumatic diseases: a challenge for cardio-rheumatology. Diagnostics (Basel). 2019;9(4):217.

42. Hinojar R, Foote L, Sangle S, Marber M, Mayr M, Carr-White G, et al. Native T1 and T2 mapping by CMR in lupus myocarditis: disease recognition and response to treatment. Int J Cardiol. 2016;222:717–726.

43. Ferreira VM, Schulz-Menger J, Holmvang G, Kramer CM, Carbone I, Sechtem U, et al. Cardiovascular magnetic resonance in non-ischemic myocardial inflammation: expert recommendations. J Am Coll Cardiol. 2018;72(24):3158–76.

44. Mavrogeni S, Gargani L, Pepe A, Monti L, Markousis-Mavrogenis G, De Santis M, et al. Cardiac magnetic resonance predicts ventricular arrhythmias in scleroderma: the Scleroderma Arrhythmia Clinical Utility Study (SAnCtUS). Rheumatology. 2020;59(8):1938–1948.

45. Rosmini S, Seraphim A, Knott K, Brown JT, Knight DS, Zaman S, et al. Non-invasive characterization of pleural and pericardial effusions using T1 mapping by magnetic resonance imaging. Eur Heart J Cardiovasc Imaging. 2022;23(8):1117–1126.

46. Cremer PC, Tariq MU, Karwa A, Alraies MC, Benatti R, Schuster A, et al. Quantitative assessment of pericardial delayed hyperenhancement predicts clinical improvement in patients with constrictive pericarditis treated with anti-inflammatory therapy. Circ Cardiovasc Imaging. 2015;8(5):e003125.

47. Baptista R, Serra S, Martins R, Teixeira R, Castro G, Salvador MJ, et al. Exercise echocardiography for the assessment of pulmonary hypertension in systemic sclerosis: a systematic review. Arthritis Res Ther. 2016;18(1):153.

48. Shaikh F, Anklesaria Z, Shagroni T, Saggar R, Gargani L, Bossone E, et al. A review of exercise pulmonary hypertension in systemic sclerosis. J Scleroderma Relat Disord. 2019;4(3):225–237.

49. Manchanda AS, Kwan AC, Ishimori M, Thomson LEJ, Li D, Berman DS, et al. Coronary microvascular dysfunction in patients with systemic lupus erythematosus and chest pain. Front Cardiovasc Med. 2022;9:867155.

50. Kwong RY, Ge Y, Steel K, Bingham S, Abdullah S, Fujikura K, et al. Cardiac magnetic resonance stress perfusion imaging for evaluation of patients with chest pain. J Am Coll Cardiol. 2019;74(14):1741–1755.

51. Thomson LE, Wei J, Agarwal M, Haft-Baradaran A, Shufelt C, Mehta PK, et al. Cardiac magnetic resonance myocardial perfusion reserve index is reduced in women with coronary microvascular dysfunction. A National Heart, Lung, and

Blood Institute-sponsored study from the Women's Ischemia Syndrome Evaluation. Circ Cardiovasc Imaging. 2015;8(4). https://doi.org/10.1161/CIRCIMAGING.114.002481

52. Zhou W, Lee JCY, Leung ST, Lai A, Lee TF, Chiang JB, et al. Long-term prognosis of patients with coronary microvascular disease using stress perfusion cardiac magnetic resonance. JACC Cardiovasc Imaging. 2021;14(3):602–611.

53. Ishimori ML, Martin R, Berman DS, Goykhman P, Shaw LJ, Shufelt C, et al. Myocardial ischemia in the absence of obstructive coronary artery disease in systemic lupus erythematosus. JACC Cardiovasc Imaging. 2011;4(1):27–33.

54. Sandhu VK, Wei J, Thomson LEJ, Berman DS, Schapira J, Wallace D, et al. Five-year follow-up of coronary microvascular dysfunction and coronary artery disease in systemic lupus erythematosus: results from a community-based lupus cohort. Arthritis Care Res (Hoboken). 2020;72(7):882–887.

55. Chen MT, Chang J, Manchanda AS, Cook-Wiens G, Shufelt CL, Anderson RD, et al. Autoimmune rheumatic diseases in women with coronary microvascular dysfunction: a report from the Women's Ischemia Syndrome Evaluation-Coronary Vascular Dysfunction (WISE-CVD) project. Front Cardiovasc Med. 2023;10:1155914.

56. Arnett DK, Blumenthal RS, Albert MA, Buroker AB, Goldberger ZD, Hahn EJ, et al. 2019 ACC/AHA guideline on the primary prevention of cardiovascular disease: a report of the American College of Cardiology/American Heart Association Task Force on Clinical Practice Guidelines. J Am Coll Cardiol. 2019;74(10):e177–e232.

57. Martinez-Ceballos MA, Sinning Rey JC, Alzate-Granados JP, Mendoza-Pinto C, Garcia-Carrasco M, Montes-Zabala L, et al. Coronary calcium in autoimmune diseases: a systematic literature review and meta-analysis. Atherosclerosis. 2021;335:68–76.

58. Andreini D, Magnoni M, Conte E, Masson S, Mushtaq S, Berti S, et al. Coronary plaque features on CTA can identify patients at increased risk of cardiovascular events. JACC Cardiovasc Imaging. 2020;13(8):1704–1717.

59. Conte E, Annoni A, Pontone G, Mushtaq S, Guglielmo M, Baggiano A, et al. Evaluation of coronary plaque characteristics with coronary computed tomography angiography in patients with non-obstructive coronary artery disease: a long-term follow-up study. Eur Heart J Cardiovasc Imaging. 2017;18(10):1170–1178.

60. Patel MR, Norgaard BL, Fairbairn TA, Nieman K, Akasaka T, Berman DS, et al. 1-year impact on medical practice and clinical outcomes of FFR(CT): the ADVANCE Registry. JACC Cardiovasc Imaging. 2020;13(1 Pt 1): 97–105.

61. Kronzer VL, Tarabochia AD, Lobo Romero AS, Tan NY, O'Byrne TJ, Crowson CS, et al. Lack of association of spontaneous coronary artery dissection with autoimmune disease. J Am Coll Cardiol. 2020;76(19):2226–2234.

62. Reynolds HR, Maehara A, Kwong RY, Sedlak T, Saw J, Smilowitz NR, et al. Coronary optical coherence tomography and cardiac magnetic resonance imaging to determine underlying causes of myocardial infarction with nonobstructive coronary arteries in women. Circulation. 2021;143(7):624–640.

63. AlBadri A, Bairey Merz CN, Johnson BD, Wei J, Mehta PK, Cook-Wiens G, et al. Impact of abnormal coronary reactivity on long-term clinical outcomes in women. J Am Coll Cardiol. 2019;73(6):684–693.

64. Seitz A, Gardezy J, Pirozzolo G, Probst S, Athanasiadis A, Hill S, et al. Long-term follow-up in patients with stable angina and unobstructed coronary arteries undergoing intracoronary acetylcholine testing. JACC Cardiovasc Interv. 2020;13(16):1865–1876.

65. Gornik HL, Creager MA. Aortitis. Circulation. 2008;117(23): 3039–3051.

66. Bois JP, Anand V, Anavekar NS. Detection of inflammatory aortopathies using multi-modality imaging. Circ Cardiovasc Imaging. 2019;12(7):e008471.

67. Roman MJ, Salmon JE. Cardiovascular manifestations of rheumatologic diseases. Circulation. 2007;116(20):2346–2355.

68. Meini S, De Franco V, Auteri A, Pieragalli D. Images in cardiovascular medicine. Takayasu's arteritis: the "macaroni sign". Circulation. 2006;114(16):e544.

69. Litmanovich DE, Yildirim A, Bankier AA. Insights into imaging of aortitis. Insights Imaging. 2012;3(6):545–560.

70. Liu M, Liu W, Li H, Shu X, Tao X, Zhai Z. Evaluation of takayasu arteritis with delayed contrast-enhanced MR imaging by a free-breathing 3D IR turbo FLASH. Medicine. 2017;96(51):e9284.

3

Rheumatoid arthritis

DIANA YANG AND MARVEN GEREL CABLING

INTRODUCTION

Rheumatoid arthritis (RA) is one of the most common autoimmune conditions with a prevalence of 0.5–1% in the United States and northern Europe (1,2). While generally known for affecting the joints, RA is a systemic disease and can also affect various other organs including, but not limited to, the ocular, pulmonary, and cardiovascular systems.

RA is diagnosed based on a combination of patient symptoms, laboratory tests, and imaging findings. The 2010 American College of Rheumatology (ACR) classification criteria for RA include scoring for joint involvement with subsets for small vs. large joints and a number of involved joints (Table 3.1). The classification criteria also include points for the following labs: C-reactive protein (CRP), erythrocyte sedimentation rate (ESR), rheumatoid factor (RF), and anti-cyclic citrullinated peptide (CCP) antibodies. Finally, there is a section of the criteria that addresses the duration of symptoms (3). However, as the criteria are used to identify patients for research, not all patients with RA fit the classification criteria and not all patients who fit the classification criteria necessarily have RA. It is important to note that, to use the criteria, the patient should have definite swelling (synovitis) in at least one joint and other diagnoses that could better account for the symptoms must be ruled out. Still, the points included in the classification criteria can provide a starting point for potentially helpful information when evaluating to see if a patient may have RA.

As mentioned, diagnosing RA requires a combination of information and often begins with an assessment of the patient's symptoms. Inflammatory joint pain is often key in the diagnosis and is described as joint pain that is worse with rest and better with activity. This may manifest with symptoms of morning stiffness where patients feel the need to "warm up" the joints after waking up. In some cases, this stiffness can be persistent throughout the day. Notable laboratory tests for RA include inflammatory markers (CRP and ESR), RF, anti-CCP antibodies, and anti-carbamylated protein antibodies. Various imaging modalities may also be helpful in diagnosis and disease monitoring. X-rays are commonly used as the initial imaging modality, though early-stage disease often does not display evident joint erosion. Musculoskeletal ultrasound is emerging as a helpful tool in visualizing synovitis and can provide useful insights when assessing a patient for inflammatory arthritis (4).

RA is treated with a variety of disease-modifying antirheumatic drugs (DMARDs). DMARDs can be divided into conventional synthetic, targeted synthetic, and biologic DMARDs. Initial treatment may include steroid medications, such as prednisone, due to their more rapid onset of action compared to other available treatments. First-line treatment typically entails initiating a conventional synthetic DMARD, such as methotrexate. If this is inadequate in reducing disease activity, a conventional synthetic DMARD, biologic DMARD, or targeted synthetic DMARD is

DOI: 10.1201/9781003386711-3

Table 3.1 ACR/EULAR 2010 classification criteria for rheumatoid arthritis

Domain	Category	Point score
A	Joint involvement	
	1 large joint	0
	2–10 large joints	1
	1–3 small joints	2
	4–10 small joints	3
	>10 joints including at least one small joint	5
B	Serology	
	Negative RF and negative ACPA	0
	Low positive RF or low positive ACPA	2
	High positive RF or high positive ACPA	3
C	Acute-phase reactants	
	Normal CRP and normal ESR	0
	Abnormal CRP or abnormal ESR	1
D	Duration of symptoms	
	<6 weeks	0
	≥6 weeks	1

Source: Adapted from Aletaha et al. (3).

Note: The points from each domain are added together for a total score. A total score of ≥6 is needed to classify a patient as having definite rheumatoid arthritis.

added. Other conventional synthetic DMARD treatment options include leflunomide, sulfasalazine, and hydroxychloroquine. The biologic DMARD category includes a growing variety of drugs that target various cytokines and other immune system processes. These include inhibitors of tumor necrosis factor (TNF) (adalimumab, certolizumab, etanercept, infliximab, golimumab), interleukin (IL)-6 (tocilizumab, sarilumab), IL-1 (anakinra), CD80/86 co-stimulation (abatacept), and CD20 (rituximab). Targeted synthetic DMARDs, such as baricitinib, tofacitinib, and upadacitinib, are all small molecules that specifically inhibit the Janus kinase (JAK) pathway to exert its effects. The choice of treatment may depend on the specific organ systems affected, certain treatments may be more beneficial or harmful, and some treatments may have more robust treatment data than others.

RA not only affects the joints but also has extra-articular manifestations that are observed in up to 50% of patients with RA (5). The cardiovascular system is among the organ systems affected. For the purpose of this chapter, we will focus on the various cardiac manifestations of RA, touching on the various vascular, pericardial, myocardial,

valvular, and conduction abnormalities that are observed.

Atherosclerosis in rheumatoid arthritis

One of the prominent impacts of RA on the cardiovascular system is the promotion of atherosclerotic disease through inflammation. The effect of RA on cardiovascular health can be as significant as that of traditional risk factors for cardiovascular disease. However, this effect is often overlooked and not incorporated into most cardiovascular risk scoring systems. Surprisingly, approximately 50% of deaths in patients with RA are attributable to cardiovascular causes (6). Moreover, patients with seropositive RA tend to develop cardiovascular disease at a younger age. Another notable aspect is that patients with RA may not exhibit typical symptoms of myocardial infection (MI). Rather, they may present with atypical symptoms and are less likely to report anginal symptoms (7).

Inflammation has been identified as a key factor associated with atherosclerotic disease. However, the exact relationship between inflammation and atherosclerosis remains partially understood, and it is uncertain whether inflammation is a consequence, cause, or parallel process to atherosclerosis. Nonetheless, research has demonstrated that both RA and atherosclerosis involve similar mechanisms and share common cytokines, such as IL-1, IL-6, and TNF (8). IL-6 and TNFα, in particular, have been found to correlate with atherosclerosis independently of other cardiovascular risk factors (9). Additional inflammatory markers, including CRP and fibrinogen, also appear to be involved in the development of atherosclerosis. The effects of these inflammatory molecules extend beyond vessel-related effects, such as endothelial dysfunction, and can influence other associated risk factors like lipid levels and insulin resistance. Paradoxically, the inflammation associated with RA is inversely associated with lipid levels such that increased inflammation (reflected by higher CRP and IL-6 levels) is linked to lower lipid levels (10). The association between elevated inflammatory markers and cardiovascular disease was investigated in a study involving elderly patients aged 70–79 years. The participants were divided into three groups based on their cardiovascular health status: Those with diagnosed cardiovascular disease, those with subclinical cardiovascular disease (defined as positive findings on the Rose questionnaire, an ankle-brachial index <0.9, or abnormal EKG findings), and those without cardiovascular disease. Blood levels of inflammatory markers were measured, with IL-6 and TNFα showing the most significant findings. The odds ratio for elevated IL-6 in subclinical cardiovascular disease was 1.58 (95% confidence interval [CI] 1.26 to 1.97), while the odds ratio for elevated TNFα in subclinical cardiovascular disease was 1.48 (95% CI 1.16–1.88). In clinical cardiovascular disease, the odds ratio for elevated IL-6 was 2.35 (95% CI 1.79–3.09), and for elevated TNFα, it was 2.05 (95% CI 1.55–2.72) (8).

IL-1β has been identified as a potential target for the treatment of atherosclerotic disease due to its involvement in the inflammatory pathway (11). Factors such as cholesterol crystals, disturbances in blood flow (known as atheroprone flow), and local tissue hypoxia can activate the NLRP3 inflammasome (12). This, in turn, triggers the release of IL-1β, which leads to endothelial inflammation and the development of atherosclerosis. In a clinical trial called the Canakinumab Anti-Inflammatory Thrombosis Outcomes Study (CANTOS), the effectiveness of canakinumab, an IL-1β inhibitor, as a potential treatment for atherosclerotic disease was evaluated (13). The trial spanned 48 months and enrolled patients with a prior myocardial infarction (MI) and elevated levels of high sensitivity CRP (2 mg/L or more) despite undergoing other methods of secondary prevention. The patients were assigned to receive a placebo, 50, 150, or 300 mg of intravenous canakinumab as a loading dose (administered every 2 weeks for 2 doses), followed by maintenance doses every 3 months. The primary endpoint was the occurrence of a non-fatal MI, stroke, or cardiovascular death. Secondary endpoints included hospitalization for unstable angina leading to urgent revascularization and the incidence of new-onset diabetes. The results indicated a potential benefit in the 150-mg canakinumab group. The hazard ratio for the primary endpoint comparing the 150-mg canakinumab group to the placebo group was 0.85 (p=0.02075). For the secondary endpoint of hospitalization for unstable angina requiring urgent revascularization, the hazard ratio was 0.83 (p=0.00525). Although some of the other endpoints showed lower rates of occurrence compared to the placebo group, they did not reach statistical significance.

IL-6 is another potential target for intervention, as it acts downstream from IL-1β and mediates various effects. For instance, CRP promotes blood clotting on the vascular endothelium, and IL-6 plays a role in promoting CRP synthesis in the liver. IL-6 also promotes platelet production (14). Furthermore, IL-6 is involved in the development of insulin resistance, which contributes to the development of type 2 diabetes mellitus—a recognized major cardiovascular risk factor (15). Interestingly, while IL-6 inhibition is an approach used in the treatment of RA, the use of anti-IL-6 agents has been associated with an increase in lipid levels (16). This paradoxical effect of inflammation from RA and lipid levels may be related. However, studies have suggested that although IL-6 inhibition does increase cholesterol levels, it does not correspondingly increase the risk of cardiovascular events (17).

TNFα and TNF receptors have been found to be upregulated in patients with heart failure (HF), and a mutation in the TNFα gene is associated with the development of coronary disease. In mice, inhibiting TNFα has been shown to reduce atherosclerosis in apolipoprotein E knockout mice (18). The role of TNFα in cardiac disease has been investigated through trials using etanercept, but no significant benefit was observed, and in some cases, there was potential for harm (19). Rheumatologists generally avoid TNF inhibitors (TNFi) in patients with uncontrolled HF, as discussed in detail later in this chapter. However, studies have indicated a decrease in cardiac events in RA patients treated with TNFi drugs, which may be attributed to the control of the underlying disease rather than the direct benefits of TNF inhibition for cardiac conditions.

The risk that RA contributes to cardiovascular disease may start even prior to the onset of symptoms of RA. One study showed that RA patients had a three times higher likelihood of hospitalization for an MI 2 years leading up to the diagnosis of RA compared to age and sex-matched individuals without RA. This finding was not replicated in another study with Swedish cohorts, however. On the other hand, multiple studies have found an increased risk of MI after RA diagnosis, overall suggesting a 1.5–2× increased risk.

Despite the increased risk of cardiovascular disease associated with RA, many commonly used risk calculators do not take RA into account. For instance, calculators like the Framingham risk calculator and the American College of Cardiology/American Heart Association Pooled Cohort Equation risk calculators do not include RA as a risk factor. Some other calculators have attempted to incorporate RA risk indirectly by including inflammatory markers or directly, such as the QRISK, QRISK2, and QRISK3 calculators developed in the United Kingdom using data from the QResearch database (6, 20, 21). However, the limited inclusion of RA in these calculators leads to an underestimation of cardiovascular risk in RA patients. This underestimation is further compounded by the paradoxical relationship between inflammation in RA and lipid levels, where increased inflammation may be calculated as decreased risk due to lower lipid levels. Moreover, the full impact of inflammation and RA on cardiovascular risk is not yet fully understood, making it challenging to accurately estimate the risk associated with RA (10). Nevertheless, recent studies suggest that the risk from RA is comparable to that of type 2 diabetes mellitus (22). Efforts to develop RA-specific cardiovascular risk calculators, such

as the ATACC-RA (TransAtlantic Cardiovascular Risk Calculator for Rheumatoid Arthritis) and ERS-RA (Expanded Risk Score in Rheumatoid Arthritis), have shown limited predictive ability for cardiovascular events. Additionally, regional differences in cardiovascular risk further complicate risk estimation. As a solution to these limitations, the European Alliance of Associations for Rheumatology (EULAR) currently recommends using general population risk calculators and applying a multiplication factor of 1.5 for RA patients (23).

Furthermore, RA exacerbates the outcomes of patients who have both RA and cardiovascular disease. The increased mortality associated with cardiovascular disease in RA patients does not occur immediately after the onset of RA symptoms but rather several years later (6) The estimated increase in cardiovascular disease mortality for RA patients compared to the general population is around 50% (6). Specifically, RA patients who experience an MI have a 1.5 times higher risk of recurrent ischemia and long-term mortality compared to non-RA patients (24). RA also elevates the risk of all types of strokes, with a risk ratio of 1.91 (95% CI, 1.73–2.12) (6). Some of this increased risk is attributed to a higher likelihood of atrial fibrillation and valvular disease, in addition to atherosclerotic disease. Additionally, RA patients should be monitored for HF, as it affects treatment options, as previously mentioned in relation to TNF inhibitors, and RA patients are more prone to developing HF.

Cardiac dysfunction and heart failure

HF affects approximately 6 million adults in the United States, which accounts for around 1.8% of the population (25). Within this population, approximately half of the cases are classified as HF with reduced ejection fraction (HFrEF), while the other half are categorized as HF with preserved ejection fraction (HFpEF) (25). In patients with RA, HFpEF is the more predominant subtype (26).

RA patients have a twofold higher risk of developing HF compared to the general population (27). This increased risk is associated with excess mortality and ranks as the second leading cause of death in RA patients, following coronary artery disease (28). The higher incidence of both ischemic and non-ischemic heart disease in RA patients, which are established risk factors for HF, contributes to this elevated risk. However, even in the absence of ischemia, HF occurs more frequently in RA patients (29). The presence of hypertension, ischemic heart disease, and other traditional cardiovascular risk factors does not fully explain this increased risk (30). It is reasonable to propose that RA itself acts as an independent risk factor for the development of HF. The combination of systemic inflammation and the existing burden of risk factors in RA patients synergistically increases cardiac morbidity in this population.

HF is not solely a late complication of RA; it can manifest even in the early stages of the disease. Two cohorts from Sweden have demonstrated a rapid increase in the risk of HF, particularly non-ischemic HF, shortly after RA diagnosis. The severity of RA disease activity is associated with all types of HF, but it is more pronounced in non-ischemic HF (29). Furthermore, a study utilizing an English primary care database found an excess risk of stroke and HF in early-stage RA. The risk is 1.4-fold higher even in the 5 years preceding the RA diagnosis, and the risk persists thereafter (31).

The chronic inflammation observed in RA significantly contributes to the heightened risk of developing HF. Among RA patients, elevated inflammatory markers such as ESR and CRP are associated with a higher risk, suggesting a direct link between inflammation and cardiac dysfunction (26). Advanced imaging studies, including cardiac magnetic resonance imaging (cMRI) and 18-fluorodeoxyglucose positron emission tomography with computed tomography (FDG-PET/CT), have provided evidence of myocardial abnormalities and inflammation in RA patients. In one study, cMRI was conducted on a group of RA patients with no known cardiac disease, revealing myocardial alterations and delayed enhancement in 45% of the patients. These findings were associated with higher RA disease activity (32). Similarly, FDG-PET/CT studies have shown that subclinical myocardial inflammation is common in RA patients and is also correlated with higher inflammatory activity (33).

The use of anti-inflammatory medications in patients with active RA has been associated with a lower risk of HF, highlighting the role of inflammation in driving HF (26). Methotrexate use has been shown to reduce cardiovascular mortality and decrease the risk of HF in RA patients over a period of 3–4 years (34). However, the Cardiovascular Inflammation Reduction Trial (CIRT), which studied a population without RA, did not demonstrate this protective effect. In this randomized controlled trial, methotrexate was compared to placebo in non-RA patients with coronary artery disease or previous MI, along with either diabetes mellitus or metabolic syndrome. The study was stopped early as there was no improvement in cardiovascular risk or inflammatory markers such as IL-1, IL-6, and CRP levels with the use of methotrexate (35). The absence of cardiovascular protection from methotrexate in the CIRT study may be attributed to the lower inflammatory levels observed in the population studied compared to those with RA. This contrasts with the findings of the CANTOS trial mentioned earlier, where canakinumab, when added to optimal medical therapy, effectively prevented adverse cardiac events (35).

The use of TNFi drugs in improving cardiac function in patients with HF has been investigated. The proposed mechanism is that TNF cytokines may contribute to the progression of HF, as chronic TNF overstimulation leads to increased levels of pro-inflammatory cytokines, including IL-1β and IL-6. This impairs β-adrenergic receptor response, resulting in systolic dysfunction, cardiac hypertrophy, and induction of cardiomyocyte apoptosis in patients with HF (36). Therefore, inhibiting TNF is thought to improve the course of the disease. Two trials were conducted using etanercept, a TNFi, to evaluate this hypothesis. However, both trials were terminated due to futility and lack of efficacy. Furthermore, one of the trials suggested higher mortality in the etanercept-treated group compared to placebo (37). Similar findings were observed in subsequent studies using another TNFi, infliximab, where a short course of infliximab at 5 mg/kg or 10 mg/kg on weeks 0, 2, and 6 did not improve outcomes and the higher dose increased the risk of death (hazard ratio 2.84) (38). As a result, prescribing labels now include caution regarding the use of this class of medication in patients with HF. Infliximab at doses >5 mg/kg is contraindicated in patients with moderate or severe HF. While TNFi may exacerbate HF and lead to negative outcomes, the use of lower doses and in patients with milder HF appears to be well-tolerated. Nonetheless, multiple studies continue to demonstrate the benefits of TNFi in reducing the overall risk of cardiovascular events.

A systematic review has shown that TNFi therapy is associated with a reduced risk of all cardiovascular events, MI, and cerebrovascular accidents (39). When compared in cross-sectional studies, there is no significant difference in the prevalence of HF between patients treated with TNFi and those treated with non-TNFi medications (40).

Cardiac arrhythmias and conduction disturbances

RA is associated with rhythm and conduction abnormalities, which are important cardiac manifestations of the disease. Malignant arrhythmias can occur in RA and may lead to sudden cardiac death. Additionally, tachyarrhythmias such as atrial fibrillation, atrial flutter, and ventricular tachycardias are more common in patients with rheumatologic disorders, including RA.

As mentioned earlier, both ischemic heart disease and HF are increased in RA, and atherosclerotic coronary artery disease is more prevalent in this population, which can result in acute coronary syndrome and ventricular arrhythmias (41). These factors contribute to the heightened risk of arrhythmias in RA. Structural changes associated with HF and ischemic heart disease are known to promote arrhythmic risk, both in RA and the general population. Furthermore, the infiltration of mononuclear cells or rheumatoid granuloma into the atrioventricular node and other conducting tissues is believed to be a primary cause of conduction abnormalities in RA (42).

Patients with RA have more than twice the risk of sudden cardiac death compared to those without RA, as demonstrated in a population-based study conducted over 15 years (7). Importantly, this increased risk of sudden cardiac death persisted even after adjusting for factors such as a history of hospitalized or unrecognized MI and revascularization procedures. This highlights that factors related to systemic inflammation contribute to the elevated risk of arrhythmias in RA. It has been observed that most conduction disorders occur during active disease in patients with autoimmune rheumatic conditions (41). There are likely additive and negative effects of non-structural inflammation-driven influences on the conduction system, leading to a higher risk of arrhythmias and contributing to the increased cardiovascular morbidity and mortality in this population. Therefore, it is reasonable to conclude that reducing the systemic inflammatory burden through tight disease control could lower the risk of arrhythmias and prevent associated complications (43).

Valvular heart disease

Valvular heart disease (VHD) is commonly found in patients with RA, with prevalence rates ranging from 83% to 97% (44, 45). These abnormalities can manifest as valve thickening or nodules, valve insufficiency, mitral valve prolapse, aortic root abnormalities, and others (45, 46). Most of the valve abnormalities observed are subclinical, typically affecting a single valve, with the mitral valve being the most commonly involved. VHD is often incidentally detected during echocardiography or focused physical examination.

Studies utilizing transesophageal echocardiography (TEE) in RA patients have shown that the lesions primarily affect the left-sided valves, with valve thickening (53%) and valve nodules (32%) being the most common findings (45). A systematic review with meta-analysis of case–control studies using echocardiography revealed that tricuspid valve insufficiency, aortic valve stenosis, and mitral valve thickening or calcification are five times more prevalent in RA patients compared to controls. Other valvular alterations, including aortic valve thickening and mitral valve insufficiency, are increased four and three times, respectively, in RA patients (47).

The development of VHD in RA does not appear to correlate with disease activity or clinical and laboratory parameters of RA (45). It is important to note that VHD in the general population is associated with increased cardiovascular morbidity and mortality (48). Mitral annular calcifications have been identified as an independent risk factor for incident cardiovascular disease and death, both in the general population and in RA patients, where valvular calcifications may predict premature atherosclerosis (49, 50). Additionally, clinically apparent VHD in RA can be complicated by thromboembolism, valvulitis, rupture of nodules, or infective endocarditis (45).

While most VHD in RA remains asymptomatic, symptomatic disease can occur, particularly due to valve incompetence. Valvulitis, inflammation of the cardiac valves and surrounding tissues, has been documented as a consequence of RA, although it is rare and its true prevalence is unknown. There have been reported cases of RA-related valvulitis, such as mitral valvulitis and aortic valve involvement, where patients presented with symptoms such as dyspnea, heart block, or severe HF (51, 52). Advanced imaging techniques, including cMRI, FDG-PET/CT, and echocardiography, have demonstrated inflammatory activity on the affected valves and surrounding structures. Surgical intervention, such as valve replacement, may be required in severe cases. These cases of valvulitis were associated with high inflammatory RA disease activity, which contrasts with most cases of VHD in RA that are asymptomatic and incidentally discovered. Due to the relative rarity of symptomatic VHD in RA, there are no formal recommendations for screening and treatment. Maintaining a high index of suspicion and conducting a focused physical examination, considering imaging when appropriate, can aid in the diagnosis of VHD in RA patients.

Rheumatoid nodules

Rheumatoid nodules, although most commonly found in the skin, can also occur in the heart as a manifestation of RA. The characterization of cutaneous rheumatoid nodules was first described in 1937 by Collins, with further details provided by Bennett, Zeller, and Bauer in 1940. These nodules typically exhibit a central area of fibrinoid necrosis surrounded by densely packed mesenchymal cells (53).

Cases of cardiac rheumatoid nodules have been documented in postmortem series and echocardiographic studies. Autopsy studies have shown a frequency of 5% for fibrinoid granulomas in various areas of the heart, with the majority of cases being asymptomatic and undetected prior to death (54). TEE studies conducted by Roldan et al have revealed valvular nodules in 32% of RA volunteers (45). However, the presence of cardiac nodules did not show a correlation with clinical or laboratory variables of RA.

In patients with RA, the likelihood of developing nodules on cardiac valves is more than ten times higher compared to individuals without RA (47). The mitral valve is most commonly affected, followed by the aortic, tricuspid, and pulmonary valves

in decreasing order (55). This pattern suggests that valvular trauma or stress may be the underlying cause for the development of these nodules. Since the mitral valve experiences the greatest stress, particularly during left ventricular systole, it is more frequently affected (55). However, there does not appear to be a correlation between the presence of subcutaneous nodules and intracardiac nodules (56).

Symptomatic cardiac rheumatoid nodules typically occur in individuals who have had RA for more than a decade and test positive for RF antibodies. The incidence is similar between males and females. The clinical presentation of cardiac rheumatoid nodules can vary and may include embolic phenomena, valvular dysfunction, atrial myxoma, and presumed infective endocarditis. Embolization of the nodules is possible and can lead to cerebrovascular accidents (56). Conduction abnormalities associated with rheumatoid nodules have been reported in a case series, with syncope being a possible presentation (57). Treatment options for large and symptomatic nodules may involve excision and operative repair of the affected valve (58).

Pericarditis

In patients with RA, involvement of the pericardium, particularly the presence of pericardial effusion, is the most common cardiac manifestation (46). Pericardial effusions can be observed in 30–50% of patients with RA, with a tenfold higher risk compared to individuals without RA (47, 54). However, most patients with pericardial effusions are asymptomatic, and the condition is often detected incidentally through imaging studies or postmortem examination. Echocardiography studies have categorized pericardial effusions in RA as either minimal (end-diastolic pericardial-epicardial separation up to 4 mm) or overt (end-diastolic pericardial–epicardial separation more than 4 mm) (46). Analysis of pericardial fluid typically shows similarities to rheumatoid pleural effusions, characterized by exudative fluid with low glucose, high lactate dehydrogenase, and high protein concentrations (59). In some cases, pericardial effusions may precede the development or diagnosis of arthritis, and other pericardial manifestations, such as cholesterol pericarditis, effusive–constrictive pericarditis, and cardiac tamponade, can occur in RA patients (60, 61).

Clinically evident pericarditis occurs in less than 10% of RA patients and is characterized by symptoms such as fatigue, weight loss, fever, dyspnea, pericardial pain, elevated ESR, and anemia (27, 62). Symptomatic pericarditis is more common in patients who are seropositive with the presence of RF antibodies and have other extra-articular manifestations. Unfortunately, the overall survival of patients with symptomatic pericarditis is lower compared to age-matched controls (62).

Asymptomatic RA-associated pericarditis often resolves spontaneously and can be observed without medical therapy. However, symptomatic disease typically requires treatment similar to other causes of pericarditis. Non-steroidal anti-inflammatory drugs (NSAIDs) are the mainstay of treatment, along with corticosteroids and colchicine (63, 65). The choice and dosing of NSAIDs may vary, with aspirin, ibuprofen, and indomethacin being commonly used. Corticosteroids are less preferred due to their potential adverse effects and increased recurrence risk (64). Colchicine is used as an adjunct in treating pericarditis, especially in cases of recurrent disease (65). Consideration of TNF-inhibitor related pericardial inflammation in addition to the use of such therapy for treatment of inflammation due to rheumatoid arthritis is warranted in management decisions (66, 67). Controlling the underlying inflammatory pathology in RA is crucial, and DMARDs play an integral role in reducing overall inflammation. In refractory cases of pericardial effusion, newer agents such as IL-1 inhibitors (e.g., anakinra, rilonacept) may be considered (68, 69).

Constrictive pericarditis is a rare but serious complication of RA and can lead to significant morbidity and mortality. Mortality rates have been reported as high as 100% within 2 years in RA patients with cardiac compression (70). In severe cases, treatment options such as pericardial stripping, pericardiectomy, or pericardial drainage may be necessary (71). Therefore, early diagnosis and management are crucial to improve outcomes in patients with constrictive pericarditis.

Nonbacterial thrombotic endocarditis

Nonbacterial thrombotic endocarditis (NBTE) is a rare complication of RA characterized by the presence of noninfectious vegetation on the cardiac valves. These vegetations develop in the context of valvular endothelial injury in a hypercoagulable state. Local platelet aggregation, migration of mononuclear cells, and immune complex deposition lead to the formation of a thrombus interwoven with fibrin, resulting in a sterile aggregate that is fragile and prone to embolization (72).

The diagnosis of NBTE is typically made using echocardiography, either through transesophageal or transthoracic methods. In the past, patients were often diagnosed postmortem or intraoperatively during cardiac surgery before the availability of echocardiographic techniques (73). The vegetations seen in NBTE are typically small, broad-based, and irregular, with abscesses and valve rupture being uncommon (74). A high level of suspicion is required for diagnosis, particularly in patients with cardiac vegetation who do not show improvement despite appropriate antibiotic treatment or those with a history of thromboembolic events (75). It is crucial to rule out infection by performing serial blood cultures to differentiate NBTE from infective endocarditis.

NBTE is a rare condition, with approximately 80% of cases associated with advanced malignancy. Other underlying conditions such as systemic lupus erythematosus and antiphospholipid antibody syndrome can also be linked to NBTE, albeit less frequently. Patients with RA can develop NBTE as well (72). The most common presentations of NBTE are stroke (54%), shortness of breath (15.3%), and chest pain (11.7%). The overall prognosis is generally poor, with neurocognitive effects contributing to morbidity and recurrent embolization, underlying malignancy, or connective tissue disease leading to mortality. In one series from the Mayo Clinic, 33.3% of patients died within 1 year of NBTE diagnosis (73).

The treatment approach for NBTE involves two main aspects: Systemic anticoagulation to prevent recurrent embolization and management of the underlying cause. This may include treatment for the associated malignancy or addressing the underlying inflammatory process in cases of connective tissue disease.

CONCLUSION

Numerous studies have indicated that individuals with RA have an elevated risk of cardiovascular disease and experience poorer cardiovascular outcomes compared to the general population. This raises the question of how to address this increased risk. One crucial aspect of risk reduction is effectively managing RA and its associated inflammation. The specific type of medication used, whether conventional synthetic, targeted synthetic, or biologic DMARDs, is not as important as ensuring that the disease is appropriately treated. However, it may be prudent to avoid JAK inhibitors whenever possible in patients with significant cardiovascular disease, as they carry a black box warning for increased cardiovascular risk compared to TNFi medications. Nonetheless, it remains unclear whether this increased risk is greater than that of untreated RA.

The EULAR recommends screening for atherosclerotic disease in all patients with RA, including those who are asymptomatic. Additionally, EULAR recommends screening for cardiovascular risk factors in RA patients every 5 years. If other risk factors are identified, appropriate treatment of those risk factors is advised. This may involve optimizing blood pressure control, initiating statin therapy, and optimizing glycemic control in individuals with diabetes. It is worth noting that there are specific recommendations to use fluvastatin, pravastatin, and rosuvastatin with tocilizumab due to potential drug interactions. Close monitoring is also recommended when initiating statin therapy in combination with methotrexate, as both medications can have hepatotoxic effects. Furthermore, there are suggestions for statin and/or fibrate usage to mitigate concerns regarding myopathy, such as initiating therapy at a low dose and separating the doses of statins and fibrates if both are prescribed. However, it should be noted that these recommendations are not specific to RA patients.

Overall improvements in reducing mortality associated with cardiovascular disease have led to better outcomes for RA patients with cardiovascular complications. Nevertheless, the increased cardiovascular risk associated with RA and the development of atherosclerosis remains significant. Therefore, it is crucial to consider this heightened risk when treating patients with RA. Managing both the RA disease itself and any concurrent cardiovascular risk factors is essential to effectively mitigate cardiovascular risk and improve patient outcomes.

REFERENCES

1. Myasoedova E, Crowson CS, Kremers HM, et al. Is the incidence of rheumatoid arthritis rising?: Results from Olmsted County, Minnesota, 1955-2007. *Arthritis Rheum* 2010; 62: 1576–1582.
2. Hunter TM, Boytsov NN, Zhang X, et al. Prevalence of rheumatoid arthritis in the United States adult population in healthcare claims databases, 2004–2014. *Rheumatol Int* 2017; 37: 1551–1557.
3. Aletaha D, Neogi T, Silman AJ, et al. 2010 Rheumatoid arthritis classification criteria: An American College of Rheumatology/ European League Against Rheumatism collaborative initiative. *Arthritis Rheum* 2010; 62: 2569–2581.
4. Di Matteo A, Mankia K, Azukizawa M, et al. The role of musculoskeletal ultrasound in the rheumatoid arthritis continuum. *Curr Rheumatol Rep* 2020; 22: 41.
5. Myasoedova E, Crowson CS, Turesson C, et al. Incidence of extraarticular rheumatoid arthritis in Olmsted County, Minnesota, in 1995–2007 versus 1985–1994: A population-based study. *J Rheumatol* 2011; 38: 983–989.
6. Semb AG, Ikdahl E, Wibetoe G, et al. Atherosclerotic cardiovascular disease prevention in rheumatoid arthritis. *Nat Rev Rheumatol* 2020; 16: 361–379.
7. Maradit-Kremers H, Crowson CS, Nicola PJ, et al. Increased unrecognized coronary heart disease and sudden deaths in rheumatoid arthritis: A population-based cohort study. *Arthritis Rheum* 2005; 52: 402–411.
8. Cesari M, Penninx BWJH, Newman AB, et al. Inflammatory markers and cardiovascular disease (The Health, Aging and Body Composition [Health ABC] Study). *Am J Cardiol* 2003; 92: 522–528.
9. Rho YH, Chung CP, Oeser A, et al. Inflammatory mediators and premature coronary atherosclerosis in rheumatoid arthritis. *Arthritis Rheum* 2009; 61: 1580–1585.
10. Choy E, Ganeshalingam K, Semb AG, et al. Cardiovascular risk in rheumatoid arthritis: Recent advances in the understanding of the pivotal role of inflammation, risk predictors and the impact of treatment. *Rheumatology* 2014; 53: 2143–2154.

11. Ridker PM. From c-reactive protein to interleukin-6 to interleukin-1: Moving upstream to identify novel targets for atheroprotection. *Circ Res* 2016; 118: 145–156.

12. Abe J, Berk BC. Atheroprone flow activation of the sterol regulatory element binding protein 2 and nod-like receptor protein 3 inflammasome mediates focal atherosclerosis. *Circulation* 2013; 128: 579–582.

13. Ridker PM, Everett BM, Thuren T, et al. Antiinflammatory therapy with canakinumab for atherosclerotic disease. *N Engl J Med* 2017; 377: 1119–1131.

14. Tanaka T, Narazaki M, Kishimoto T. IL-6 in inflammation, immunity, and disease. *Cold Spring Harb Perspect Biol* 2014; 6: a016295–a016295.

15. Rehman K, Akash MSH, Liaqat A, et al. Role of interleukin-6 in development of insulin resistance and type 2 diabetes mellitus. *Crit Rev Eukaryot Gene Expr* 2017; 27: 229–236.

16. Pierini FS, Botta E, Soriano ER, et al. Effect of tocilizumab on LDL and HDL characteristics in patients with rheumatoid arthritis. An observational study. *Rheumatol Ther* 2021; 8: 803–815.

17. Castagné B, Viprey M, Martin J, et al. Cardiovascular safety of tocilizumab: A systematic review and network meta-analysis. *PLoS One* 2019; 14: e0220178.

18. Brånén L, Hovgaard L, Nitulescu M, et al. Inhibition of tumor necrosis factor-α reduces atherosclerosis in apolipoprotein E knockout mice. *Arterioscler Thromb Vasc Biol* 2004; 24: 2137–2142.

19. Anker SD, Coats AJS. How to RECOVER from RENAISSANCE? The significance of the results of RECOVER, RENAISSANCE, RENEWAL and ATTACH. *Int J Cardiol* 2002; 86: 123–130.

20. Hippisley-Cox J, Coupland C, Vinogradova Y, et al. Predicting cardiovascular risk in England and Wales: Prospective derivation and validation of QRISK2. *BMJ* 2008; 336: 1475–1482.

21. Hippisley-Cox J, Coupland C, Brindle P. Development and validation of QRISK3 risk prediction algorithms to estimate future risk of cardiovascular disease: Prospective cohort study. *BMJ* 2017; 357: j2099.

22. Peters MJL, van Halm VP, Voskuyl AE, et al. Does rheumatoid arthritis equal diabetes mellitus as an independent risk factor for cardiovascular disease? A prospective study. *Arthritis Rheum* 2009; 61: 1571–1579.

23. Agca R, Heslinga SC, Rollefstad S, et al. EULAR recommendations for cardiovascular disease risk management in patients with rheumatoid arthritis and other forms of inflammatory joint disorders: 2015/2016 update. *Ann Rheum Dis* 2017; 76: 17–28.

24. McCoy SS, Crowson CS, Maradit-Kremers H, et al. Longterm outcomes and treatment after myocardial infarction in patients with rheumatoid arthritis. *J Rheumatol* 2013; 40: 605–610.

25. Virani SS, Alonso A, Aparicio HJ, et al. Heart disease and stroke statistics—2021 update: A report from the American Heart Association. *Circulation*; 143: e254–e743. DOI: 10.1161/CIR.0000000000000950.

26. Ahlers MJ, Lowery BD, Farber-Eger E, et al. Heart failure risk associated with rheumatoid arthritis–related chronic inflammation. *J Am Heart Assoc* 2020; 9: e014661.

27. Voskuyl AE. The heart and cardiovascular manifestations in rheumatoid arthritis. *Rheumatology* 2006; 45: iv4–iv7.

28. Johnson TM, Yang Y, Roul P, et al. A narrowing mortality gap: Temporal trends of cause-specific mortality in a national matched cohort study in US veterans with rheumatoid arthritis. *Arthritis Care Res* 2023; 75(8): 1648–1658.

29. Mantel Ä, Holmqvist M, Andersson DC, et al. Association between rheumatoid arthritis and risk of ischemic and nonischemic heart failure. *J Am Coll Cardiol* 2017; 69: 1275–1285.

30. Nicola PJ, Maradit-Kremers H, Roger VL, et al. The risk of congestive heart failure in rheumatoid arthritis: A population-based study over 46 years. *Arthritis Rheum* 2005; 52: 412–420.

31. Nikiphorou E, De Lusignan S, Mallen CD, et al. Cardiovascular risk factors and outcomes in early rheumatoid arthritis: A population-based study. *Heart* 2020; 106: 1566–1572.

32. Kobayashi Y, Giles JT, Hirano M, et al. Assessment of myocardial abnormalities in rheumatoid arthritis using a comprehensive cardiac magnetic resonance approach: A pilot study. *Arthritis Res Ther* 2010; 12: R171.

33. Amigues I, Tugcu A, Russo C, et al. Myocardial inflammation, measured using 18-Fluorodeoxyglucose positron emission tomography with computed tomography, is associated with disease activity in rheumatoid arthritis. *Arthritis Rheumatol* 2019; 71: 496–506.

34. Westlake SL, Colebatch AN, Baird J, et al. The effect of methotrexate on cardiovascular disease in patients with rheumatoid arthritis: A systematic literature review. *Rheumatology (Oxford)* 2010; 49: 295–307.

35. Ridker PM, Everett BM, Pradhan A, et al. Low-dose methotrexate for the prevention of atherosclerotic events. *N Engl J Med* 2019; 380: 752–762.

36. Baoqi Y, Dan M, Xingxing Z, et al. Effect of anti-rheumatic drugs on cardiovascular disease events in rheumatoid arthritis. *Front Cardiovasc Med* 2022; 8: 812631.

37. Enbrel prescribing information, https://www.pi.amgen.com/-/media/Project/Amgen/Repository/pi-amgen-com/Enbrel/enbrel_pi.pdf 2022.

38. Chung ES, Packer M, Lo KH, et al. Randomized, double-blind, placebo-controlled, pilot trial of infliximab, a chimeric monoclonal antibody to tumor necrosis factor-α, in patients with moderate-to-severe heart failure: Results of the anti-TNF therapy against congestive heart failure (ATTACH) trial. *Circulation* 2003; 107: 3133–3140.

39. Barnabe C, Martin B-J, Ghali WA. Systematic review and meta-analysis: Anti-tumor necrosis factor α therapy and cardiovascular events in rheumatoid arthritis. *Arthritis Care Res* 2011; 63: 522–529.

40. Schau T, Gottwald M, Arbach O, et al. Increased prevalence of diastolic heart failure in patients with rheumatoid arthritis correlates with active disease, but not with treatment type. *J Rheumatol* 2015; 42: 2029–2037.

41. Seferović PM, Ristić AD, Maksimović R, et al. Cardiac arrhythmias and conduction disturbances in autoimmune rheumatic diseases. *Rheumatology* 2006; 45: iv39–iv42.

42. Gerges L, D'Angelo K, Bass D, et al. Cardiac conduction disturbances in rheumatologic disease: A cross-sectional study. *Am J Cardiovasc Dis* 2022; 12: 31–37.

43. Lazzerini PE, Capecchi PL, Laghi-Pasini F. Systemic inflammation and arrhythmic risk: Lessons from rheumatoid arthritis. *Eur Heart J* 2016; 38: 1717–1727.

44. Guedes C, Bianchi-Fior P, Cormier B, et al. Cardiac manifestations of rheumatoid arthritis: A case-control transesophageal echocardiography study in 30 patients. *Arthritis Rheum* 2001; 45: 129–135.

45. Roldan CA, DeLong C, Qualls CR, et al. Characterization of valvular heart disease in rheumatoid arthritis by transesophageal echocardiography and clinical correlates. *Am J Cardiol* 2007; 100: 496–502.

46. Corrao S, Salli' L, Arnone S, et al. Cardiac involvement in rheumatoid arthritis: Evidence of silent heart disease. *Eur Heart J* 1995; 16: 253–256.

47. Corrao S, Messina S, Pistone G, et al. Heart involvement in rheumatoid arthritis: Systematic review and meta-analysis. *Int J Cardiol* 2013; 167: 2031–2038.

48. Santangelo G, Bursi F, Faggiano A, et al. The global burden of valvular heart disease: From clinical epidemiology to management. *J Clin Med* 2023; 12: 2178.

49. Fox CS, Vasan RS, Parise H, et al. Mitral annular calcification predicts cardiovascular morbidity and mortality: The Framingham Heart Study. *Circulation* 2003; 107: 1492–1496.

50. Yiu K-H, Wang S, Mok M-Y, et al. Relationship between cardiac valvular and arterial calcification in patients with rheumatoid arthritis and systemic lupus erythematosus. *J Rheumatol* 2011; 38: 621–627.

51. Frederiksen AS, Jørgensen SH, Wiggers H, et al. Mitral valvulitis as a severe extra-articular manifestation of rheumatoid arthritis: A case report. *Eur Heart J Case Rep* 2021; 5: ytaa467.

52. Ivy K, Egbuche O, Gill S, et al. Acute on chronic severe aortic insufficiency due to rheumatoid arthritis-associated valvulitis. *Am J Cardiovasc Dis* 2021; 11: 404–409.

53. Ellman P, Cudkowicz L, Elwood JS. Widespread serous membrane involvement by rheumatoid nodules. *J Clin Pathol* 1954; 7: 239–244.

54. Bonfiglio T. Heart disease in patients with seropositive rheumatoid arthritis: A controlled autopsy study and review. *Arch Intern Med* 1969; 124: 714.

55. Chand EM, Freant LJ, Rubin JW. Aortic valve rheumatoid nodules producing clinical aortic regurgitation and a review of the literature. *Cardiovasc Pathol* 1999; 8: 333–338.

56. Vantrease A, Trabue C, Atkinson J, et al. Large endocardial rheumatoid nodules: A case report and review of the literature. *J Community Hosp Intern Med Perspect* 2017; 7: 175–177.

57. Ahern M, Lever JV, Cosh J. Complete heart block in rheumatoid arthritis. *Ann Rheum Dis* 1983; 42: 389–397.

58. Tennyson C, Kler A, Chaturvedi A, et al. Rheumatoid nodule on the anterior mitral valve leaflet. *J Card Surg* 2018; 33: 643–645.

59. Franco AE. Rheumatoid pericarditis: Report of 17 cases diagnosed clinically. *Ann Intern Med* 1972; 77: 837.

60. Levy P-Y, Corey R, Berger P, et al. Etiologic diagnosis of 204 pericardial effusions. *Medicine* 2003; 82: 385–391.

61. Movahedian M, Afzal W, Shoja T, et al. Chest pain due to pericardial effusion as initial presenting feature of rheumatoid arthritis: Case report and review of the literature. *Cardiol Res* 2017; 8: 161–164.

62. Hara KS, Ballard DJ, Ilstrup DM, et al. Rheumatoid pericarditis: Clinical features and survival. *Medicine* 1990; 69: 81–91.

63. Imazio M, Gaita F, LeWinter M. Evaluation and treatment of pericarditis: A systematic review. *JAMA* 2015; 314: 1498.

64. Imazio M, Brucato A, Cumetti D, et al. Corticosteroids for recurrent pericarditis: High versus low doses: A nonrandomized observation. *Circulation* 2008; 118: 667–671.

65. Imazio M, Belli R, Brucato A, et al. Efficacy and safety of colchicine for treatment of multiple recurrences of pericarditis (CORP-2): A multicentre, double-blind, placebo-controlled, randomised trial. *Lancet* 2014; 383: 2232–2237.

66. Edwards MH, Leak AM. Pericardial effusions on anti-TNF therapy for rheumatoid arthritis–a drug side effect or uncontrolled systemic disease? *Rheumatology* 2008; 48: 316–317.

67. Soh MC, Hart HH, Corkill M. Pericardial effusions with tamponade and visceral constriction in patients with rheumatoid arthritis on tumour necrosis factor (TNF)-inhibitor therapy. *Int J Rheum Dis* 2009; 12: 74–77.

68. Brucato A, Imazio M, Gattorno M, et al. Effect of anakinra on recurrent pericarditis among patients with colchicine resistance and corticosteroid dependence: The AIRTRIP randomized clinical trial. *JAMA* 2016; 316: 1906.

69. Klein AL, Imazio M, Cremer P, et al. Phase 3 trial of interleukin-1 trap rilonacept in recurrent pericarditis. *N Engl J Med* 2021; 384: 31–41.

70. Escalante A, Kaufman RL, Quismorio FP, et al. Cardiac compression in rheumatoid pericarditis. *Semin Arthritis Rheum* 1990; 20: 148–163.

71. Imadachi H, Imadachi S, Koga T, et al. Successful treatment of refractory cardiac tamponade due to rheumatoid arthritis using pericardial drainage. *Rheumatol Int* 2010; 30: 1103–1106.

72. Venepally NR, Arsanjani R, Agasthi P, et al. A new insight into nonbacterial thrombotic endocarditis: A systematic review of cases. *Anatol J Cardiol* 2022; 26: 743–749.

73. Quintero-Martinez JA, Hindy J-R, El Zein S, et al. Contemporary demographics, diagnostics and outcomes in non-bacterial thrombotic endocarditis. *Heart* 2022; 108: 1637–1643.

74. Asopa S, Patel A, Khan OA, et al. Nonbacterial thrombotic endocarditis. *Eur J Cardiothorac Surg* 2007; 32: 696–701.

75. Dafer RM. Neurologic complications of nonbacterial thrombotic endocarditis. In: *Handbook of Clinical Neurology*. Elsevier, pp. 135–141.

4

Spondyloarthritis

HEATHER GILLESPIE

INTRODUCTION

Spondyloarthritis refers to a closely related group of rheumatic diseases characterized by a distinct spectrum of features, including inflammatory back pain, inflammation of the sacroiliac joints, peripheral joint synovitis, and a notable association with HLA-B27. AS (AS) represents the archetypal presentation involving the axial spine, or axial spondyloarthropathy (axSpA). In 2010, diagnostic criteria were proposed for non-radiographic axSpA (nr-axSpA) as a separate yet related entity, allowing the classification of patients with spondyloarthritis even in the absence of radiographic changes in the sacroiliac joints on X-ray.[1]

Spondyloarthritis is also known for its distinctive extra-articular manifestations (EAMs), encompassing enthesitis, psoriasis, inflammatory bowel disease (IBD), anterior uveitis, and more. Psoriatic arthritis (PsA), reactive arthritis, and enteropathic arthritis fall within this classification as well. It has been postulated that chronic inflammatory diseases may contribute to the onset and progression of cardiovascular disease (CVD).

Patients with rheumatoid arthritis (RA) and other inflammatory joint diseases face an elevated risk of cardiovascular (CV) pathology, attributed not only to traditional CV risk factors but also to chronic inflammation and autoimmunity.[2] These diseases further exhibit an increased risk of premature death compared to the general population, primarily due to the heightened risk of CVD, as indicated by both an increase in all-cause mortality assessed by standardized mortality ratios (SMRs) and CVD mortality.[3] The augmented mortality rates were found to be at least two-fold higher and closely linked with disease severity.[4]

The findings of an inception cohort study involving RA patients from the 1980s and 1990s initially brought focused attention to the risk of mortality and CVD in patients with AS and PsA.[5] While studies on mortality rates in spondyloarthritis are somewhat inconclusive, there appears to be an increased prevalence of CVD in this population.

In 2006, through a cross-sectional comparative study, Han et al. established that PsA and AS, similar to RA, seem to share an increase in CV risk.[6] The study included 3,066 PsA patients and 1,843 AS patients and revealed that the prevalence for ischemic heart disease (IHD), atherosclerosis, peripheral vascular disease, congestive heart failure (CHF), cerebrovascular disease, type II diabetes (DM), hyperlipidemia, and hypertension (HTN) was higher in RA compared to the PsA and AS. However, PsA demonstrated significantly increased rates in all listed comorbidities of CVD (except atherosclerosis), as did AS (except atherosclerosis and DM). While the data suggested that RA carried a higher risk for all these parameters more so than PsA or AS, limitations of the study included the absence of data on confounding factors like family history of heart disease, disease severity of the underlying rheumatic disease, smoking, or a previous diagnosis of CVD. Additionally, the study exclusively focused on non-fatal CVD.

DOI: 10.1201/9781003386711-4

In a prospective nationwide cohort study conducted in Sweden from 2001 to 2012, which included patients with AS, PsA, and undifferentiated spondyloarthritis (combined nearly 30,000), as well as a general population (266,435) control, researchers compared the risk for acute coronary syndrome (ACS). They found a standardized incidence ratio (SIR) of 4.3–5.4, compared to 3.2 in the general population. SIRs for stroke were also elevated, ranging from 5.4 to 5.9 compared to 4.7 in the general population, and venous thromboembolism rates were similarly elevated.[7]

PATHOPHYSIOLOGY

Atherosclerosis is known to undergo accelerated progression in chronic inflammatory rheumatic diseases. While data on AS and PsA is less extensive than in RA, there is a general consensus indicating an elevated CV risk in these patients. Apart from atherogenesis, the established role of inflammation on endothelial dysfunction in both the pathogenesis and progression of atherogenesis is well-documented.

Oxidative stress, toll-like receptor signaling, and macrophage accumulation contribute to the overexpression of proinflammatory cytokines, playing a central role in the pathophysiology of arthritides and influencing the initiation and perpetuation of the atherosclerotic process. Cytokines such as TNFα, IL1ß, and IL6 have been implicated in the atherogenic process. Alterations in lipoprotein concentrations also contribute to endothelial injury and dysfunction, activating the innate immune system, which, in turn, leads to an increase in circulating cytokines.

The manifestation of CVD, from endothelial damage and atherogenesis to plaque rupture, can also be considered an immune-mediated disease. There are notable parallels between the chronic inflammatory processes and dysregulated immune responses observed in both CVD and chronic inflammatory rheumatic diseases.[8]

ANKYLOSING SPONDYLITIS

Cardiovascular risk

In 1977, Radford and colleagues were among the pioneers in reporting an increased relative risk of CV and cerebrovascular disease, with rates of 1.3 and 1.7, respectively, in patients with spondyloarthropathy.[9] Similarly, a Scandinavian study identified spondyloarthritis as a strong predictor of early coronary bypass grafting.[10] In a Taiwanese database study, AS patients younger than 45 years old with a new diagnosis (less than 3 years of disease) demonstrated a hazard ratio (HR) of 1.44 for men with AS compared to the general population. Notably, this study did not identify an increased rate of comorbidities such as DM or HTN in the AS patients.[11] These results are consistent with findings from a cross-sectional US claims-based analysis which showed an increased risk of CHF 1.8, PVD 2.6, and CVA 1.7.[12]

Using national and population-based registers, a cohort of 5,358 AS patients, 37,245 RA patients, and 25,006 controls was examined for ACS. While the RA cohort exhibited a higher relative risk of 1.7, the rate remained elevated at 1.3 for AS patients compared to the general population.[13]

In three meta-analyses, the increased risk of myocardial infarction (MI) and stroke was found to be higher in AS patients than in controls. In 2017, Schieir et al. reported a comparable risk for incident MI across five types of arthritis. This analysis, spanning 25 articles from 1980 to 2015 and encompassing RA, PsA, AS, gout, and osteoarthritis (OA), indicated a trend toward increased risk with a relative risk of 1.24 for AS patients. However, RA, PsA, and gout retained a significantly increased MI risk even after correcting for traditional risk factors.[14]

In another meta-analysis reviewing data from more than 27,000 AS patients, a significant increase in MI was reported in AS patients, with an odds ratio (OR) of 1.6 in seven of the studies analyzed. Additionally, the risk of stroke was significantly increased with an OR of 1.5.[15] Finally, a meta-analysis from the Mayo Clinic in 2015 regarding coronary artery disease (CAD) in AS patients found an overall risk ratio of 1.41 for CAD in AS patients. This meta-analysis examined risk ratios for cross-sectional studies vs cohort studies and identified a higher risk in cross-sectional studies (2.08).[16]

In 2020, a Swedish study looked at the characteristics and mortality of AS patients hospitalized with their first acute MI (AMI) and compared them to the general population. This retrospective cohort study, spanning from 2006 to 2014, identified 292 subjects with AS with a significantly increased rate of pulmonary disease, thromboembolic disease,

DM, HTN, and renal disease as well as a higher rate of stable IHD, CHF, cerebrovascular accidents (CVA), and valvular heart disease. However, there was no difference in mortality due to CVD-related causes, though the overall mortality at 1 year was increased in AS patients vs comparators at an HR of 2. Furthermore, upon discharge, less AS patients were prescribed lipid-lowering therapy (79% vs 87%) and non-aspirin platelet therapy (63% vs 76%) compared to the general population.[17]

Mortality

Over the years, conflicting reports have emerged regarding mortality and CV risk in AS. While most studies demonstrate an increase in IHD compared to the general population and an elevated prevalence of traditional CV risk factors, not all findings align. An analysis from the Mayo Clinic in 1979 reported no significant difference in mortality between male patients with AS and the general male population.[18] However, during the same era, several studies conducted in the UK, Canada, Finland, Norway, China, and Sweden reported an SMR ranging from 1.6 to 1.9.[19]

In a study evaluating 398 hospitalized patients with AS between 1961 and 1969, the overall mortality rate was reportedly 1.5 times the expected rate.[20] Similar findings of increased mortality rates are reported in AS cohorts in Norway and Hong Kong involving 2,154 AS patients, concluded with elevated mortality rates (SMR) of 1.63 and 1.89, respectively.[21] In 2016, a nationwide cohort study of AS patients in Sweden found the adjusted HR for death to be 1.6.[22]

In a retrospective cohort study evaluating 21,473 AS patients between 1995 and 2011, the adjusted HR for vascular death was elevated at a rate of 1.36, even after accounting for baseline comorbidities such as DM, HTN, and peripheral vascular disease.[23]

Other cardiovascular manifestations of ankylosing spondylitis

There is literature suggesting an increased prevalence of valvular heart disease and conduction abnormalities in the AS population. A 1997 review from Germany revealed a significant increase in HLA-B27 positivity among men with pacemakers.

The review also identified a cardiac syndrome characterized by severe conduction system abnormalities and aortic regurgitation, with the majority of patients exhibiting both clinical findings and positive HLA-B27. Intriguingly, half of these patients had not received a rheumatic disease diagnosis.[24]

In a 2013 cross-sectional study from Sweden, conduction disturbances were identified as common, affecting approximately 10%–33% of individuals. These disturbances, particularly presenting as first-degree atrioventricular (AV) block and prolonged QRS duration, were associated with male sex and older age, but not with disease activity.[25]

A small study in 1998 recruited 44 patients with AS and 30 age- and sex-matched healthy volunteers and underwent transesophageal echocardiography. The results indicated a high prevalence of aortic root and valve disease in AS patients (82%) compared to controls (27%) (p=<0.001). Aortic root thickening and stiffness were also frequently observed in these patients. Additionally, the study identified that patients over 45 years old with more than 15 years of disease had the highest prevalence of abnormalities.[26] In a prospective nationwide study from Sweden with over 6,000 AS patients, 16,000 PsA patients, and 5,000 undifferentiated spondyloarthritis patients, risk of cardiac rhythm disturbances and aortic regurgitation were increased compared to the general population.[27] The highest incidence rates were for atrial fibrillation (AF) and pacemaker placement. A 5-year follow-up on cardiac conduction disturbances in the AS patients demonstrated first-degree AV block as the most common finding. Associations with both AS and non-AS characteristics identified with an increased risk included male sex, older age, longer symptom duration, a history of anterior uveitis, higher AS disease activity, greater waist circumference, and medication reflecting CVD.[28]

A retrospective Canadian cohort study comprising 8,616 AS patients revealed standardized prevalence ratios of 1.58 for aortic valvular and non-valvular heart disease, 1.37 for IHD, 1.34 for CHF, and 1.25 for cerebrovascular disease.[29] In a similar population-based study from the Korean national health insurance service, 14,129 patients with newly diagnosed AS were compared them to age- and sex-matched non-AS subjects. Over a 3.5-year follow-up, more AS patients developed AF (AF) at a rate of 2.32 vs 1.51 per person years for patients without AS. There was a three times higher risk for AF in patients under 40 compared to general population.[30] A cohort study of Dutch elderly patients with AS (CARDAS) found conduction disturbances were similar between AS patients and OA controls at 23% and 24%, respectively. However, the prevalence of aortic valve regurgitation was significantly higher in AS compared to the controls at a rate of 23% compared to 11%. After correcting for age, sex, and CV risk factors, AS patients had an elevated OR of 4.5.[31]

Contrary to the aforementioned studies, a singular study that conducted electrocardiograms and echocardiograms on 100 men with AS from Switzerland revealed no increase in the rates of aortic or mitral valve regurgitation or diastolic dysfunction compared to the literature among the normal population.[32] Additionally, a systematic review and meta-analysis reported a 1.8 times higher risk of AF in patients with AS compared to individuals without AS and a 3.5 times higher rate of AV block in AS patients as well. Their conclusion includes the recommendation for routine evaluations for conduction disorders.[33]

NON-RADIOGRAPHIC SPONDYLOARTHROPATHY

In 2009, classification criteria for nr-axSpA were established, and, in 2010, treatment of nr-axSpA was first acknowledged in the European League Against Rheumatism (EULAR) recommendations for managing AS. Many studies regarding mortality and CVD prior to this time made no distinction between radiographic axSpA (r-axSpA) and axSpA, respectively. Instead, these studies would have collectively labeled patients under the umbrella term "ankylosing spondylitis." Consequently, obtaining sufficient data to determine CV risk in nr-axSpA might be challenging. However, there have been a few studies that examined the comparable rates of CV risk factors between r-axSpA and nr-axSpA.

Results of the Corrona PsA/SpA registry identified 407 patients with spondyloarthropathy – 310 AS and 97 nr-axSpA. When comparing their risk of comorbidities, AS patients and nr-axSpA patients had the same rates of HTN (37%), obesity (26%), CVD (9.6%), and DM (7%).[34] Among 775 patients from two hospital centers in Massachusetts, 641 with AS and 134 with nr-axSpA, there was no difference in the prevalence of common comorbidities

such as CAD (11%), HTN (9%). This is particularly notable considering AS patients were older (54 vs 46 years for nr-axSpA), more frequently male (77% vs 64%), and had higher serum inflammatory markers (CRP 3.4 vs 2.2).[35] These findings suggest that, despite demographic and clinical differences, nr-axSpA patients share similar comorbidity burdens with those classified as having AS.

PSORIATIC ARTHRITIS

PsA is a chronic inflammatory musculoskeletal and skin disease which affects 0.3%–1% of the general population, and PsA occurs in 20%–30% of patients with psoriasis.[36] PsA is also associated with a high prevalence of EAMs and traditional CV comorbidities. Comorbidities that are associated with PsA include HTN, DM, dyslipidemia, and obesity. In 2006, Scarpa and colleagues proposed the term psoriatic disease to highlight the clinical and pathogenetic heterogeneity of PsA.[37]

Comorbidities

A meta-analysis including 39 studies with over 152,000 PsA patients found the most prevalent comorbidities were HTN (34%), metabolic syndrome (29%), obesity (27%), hyperlipidemia (24%), and CVD (19%) and that comorbidities are more common in PsA than controls and were associated with poorer quality of life and function.[38]

Mortality

Studies on whether PsA leads to higher mortality are conflicting. Where earlier studies from tertiary rheumatology centers have revealed an increase in mortality in patients with PsA compared to the general population, later studies do not support the finding of an increased risk. PsA is characterized by a high prevalence of CV comorbidities. The association of PsA and metabolic comorbidities and IHD makes it more difficult to evaluate PsA as an independent risk factor for CVD or risk of mortality.

A study investigating hospitalized patients in Canada from 1978 to 1993, 1978 to 2004, and 1978 to 2017 revealed a statistically significant increase in standardized mortality rates. Interestingly, the data from the University of Toronto PsA cohort showed elevated SMRs compared to the general population in the initial time period of 1978–1993. Follow-up studies of the same cohort over the next 40 years revealed a trend of reduction in SMRs. The SMRs were 1.89 for 1978–1986, 1.63 for 1987–1995, and 1.05 for 1996–2004.[39] A Hong Kong study spanning 1999–2008 also found an increase in mortality rates.[40]

Reviewing mortality studies in population-based cohorts also has similarly conflicting data. Large US (1970–1999), UK (1994–2010), and Danish (1998–2004) cohorts showed no increase in mortality rates. However, cohort studies from Denmark (1997–2006), Taiwan (2001–2012), and Canada (1996–2016) each showed an increased SMR ranging from 1.34 to 1.74.[41] Finally, in 2021, from Israel, spanning the period 2003–2018, including 5275 PsA patients followed for 7 years, the authors concluded no increased risk in all-cause mortality after adjustment of comorbidities. The leading cause of death was malignancy, followed by IHD, which was in line with the order of the causes of death in the general population. This study was able to include data about smoking, BMI, comorbidities, and use of treatments (conventional and biologic disease modifying antirheumatic drugs [DMARDs]).[42]

Ischemic heart disease

An inception cohort study by Ahlehoff in 2011 from Denmark was able to match and adjust variables based on age, sex, comorbidities, and medical treatments for comorbidities. In this cohort, the RR for MI was 1.74 for PsA patients, but in the age group of 18–50, it was as high as 2.23, 1.87 in ages 51–70, and no statistically significant increase in the population over 70 years old.[43] The meta-analysis by Schieir et al., which reviewed 25 articles, published between 1985 and 2000 identified an increased relative risk of MI of 1.41 in PsA patients even after adjusting for traditional risk factors.[14]

PSORIASIS

Psoriasis is recognized as one of the more common immune-mediated inflammatory disorders, affecting approximately 1%–3% of the US population.[44] As early as 1978, an increased risk of vascular disease in psoriasis patients at a factor of 2.2 times was recognized in a clinic-based case-control study. Since then, most studies have been large retrospective or prospective database studies. The largest prospective study published by Gelfand et al. using General Practice Research Database from 1987 to 2002 comprised prospective data collected from general practitioners in Britain and showed that after adjusting for traditional CV risk factors such as HTN, DM, and dyslipidemia, there was a slightly elevated adjusted relative risk for MI among patients with mild psoriasis and a substantially elevated adjusted relative risk among patients with severe psoriasis which was even higher in younger patients.[45] Using the same data, Kaye et al. found an increased risk of factors for CVD as well as increased rates of MI, angina, stroke, and peripheral vascular disease.[46] In 2009, using the same database, Brauchli et al. found no increased risk for MI overall, but in patients under 60 with severe disease, there was a noted increased MI risk.[47]

Retrospective studies from Sweden, Germany, and Finland documented increased rates of risk factors such as HTN, DM, and obesity in patients with psoriasis. Retrospective studies showed increased CV mortality in hospitalized patients (1.86) but not in outpatients (0.94). This suggests that more severe disease is associated with a higher risk of CVD and may not extend to patients with milder disease.[48]

In a cross-sectional study from a Spanish multicenter cohort, 888 axSpA patients were recruited with 19% having uveitis and 6.4% with IBD. All patients with EAMs had a significant increase in past CV events compared to axSpA patients without EAMs. The highest event rate was in psoriasis 9% vs 4% but also significant in any EAM 7% with a p=0.032.[49] An interesting trend within the studies of patients with psoriasis was an increased risk for all-cause mortality, and this appeared to be related to the degree of skin disease severity.

Ischemic heart disease

In a cohort study the OR of developing MI in patients with psoriasis less than 60 years old was 1.66, though this increased risk was only found in severe, not mild, psoriasis.[45] A meta-analysis of 75 observational studies encompassing > 500,000 patients with psoriasis and > 29 million controls demonstrated an RR for CVD of 1.4 and IHD (including MI) of 1.5 in psoriasis. However, the risk of CV and cerebrovascular disease was not increased.[50] A review in 2010 provided an overview of the literature supporting the CVD risk and relevant risk factors in psoriasis and PsA looking at the literature from 1975 to 2009 and overall concluded that PsO and PsA patients have an elevated risk of developing CVD and that risk is greatest in patients with more severe disease and longer disease duration. Ultimately, the difficulty remains in determining if risk factors are caused by psoriasis or if they share a common pathogenesis.[51]

UVEITIS

Uveitis is one of the most common EAMs of AS, and the prevalence is approximately 20%–30% in AS patients. There are very limited studies on the incidence of cardiac involvement in uveitis patients; however, IHD and atherosclerosis seem to be associated with inflammatory eye disease.

In an AS population in Taiwan, collecting data spanning 15 years and including 1,181 patients with uveitis found that patients in all age groups were independently associated with an increased risk of developing AMI as compared to those without uveitis. The HR ranged from 1.55 up to 3.24 in patients over age 60 of developing AMI regardless of comorbidities.[52]

In a 2014 cross-sectional study of AS patients in Norway, of the 61% who had a history of uveitis, an increased OR was noted for HTN (3.29) and atherosclerosis (2.57) (atherosclerosis defined as having carotid plaque on ultrasound or a history of CV event).[53] A systematic review and meta-analysis, also using the Taiwanese database, largely but not exclusively AS patients with uveitis noted there was an increased risk of atherosclerosis-related CVD (AMI, ACS, and major adverse cardiac event [MACE]) by 1.49-fold.[54]

INFLAMMATORY BOWEL DISEASE (IBD)

IBD comprises two major subtypes: Crohn's disease and ulcerative colitis and characterized by chronic inflammation of the gastrointestinal tract. It is also highly associated with extraintestinal manifestations most notably an inflammatory arthritis but is also considered an EAM of spondyloarthritis.

Two retrospective cohort studies involving 17,000 and 25,000 individuals showed that the risk of MI in patients with IBD is similar to the control group.[55] However, a Danish cohort of 28,833 IBD individuals found an increased risk of CV events (RR 2.13) particularly in the first year after the IBD diagnosis.[56] Kristensen et al. found individuals with IBD had an increased risk of stroke RR 1.15 and hospitalization for heart failure RR 1.37.[57] A meta-analysis performed by Feng et al. included ten studies for review up until 2016 and included cohort studies from Sweden, Denmark, the US, Canada, the UK, and Taiwan. Patients with IBD were associated with an increased risk of IHD with a relative risk of 1.24 and was higher in females and more pronounced in younger patients.[58]

DISEASE TREATMENT AND EFFECT ON CARDIOVASCULAR EVENTS

Nonsteroidal anti-inflammatory drugs and disease modifying antirheumatic drugs

A 10-year population retrospective cohort study from Taiwan comparing 1,208 AS patients with 19,328 non-AS patients found that the use of sulfasalazine at 1,000 mg/day reduced CVD risk in patients with AS with HR of 0.65. This study also looked at celecoxib and found it was neutral regarding CVD risk in AS patients.[59] Another study demonstrated that nonsteroidal anti-inflammatory drugs and disease (NSAIDs) and statin therapy were associated with a decrease in risk for vascular mortality (HR 0.1 and HR 0.25, respectively).[23] Oza and colleagues used the UK general population database between 2000 and 2014 and compared 1,430 AS patients monitored for a mean of 5 years of follow-up and found a decrease in mortality rates in the statin users with an HR of 0.63. This appeared to be a greater benefit than what is observed in the general population or in patients with RA.[60]

A systematic review and meta-analysis performed at Mayo Clinic, which reviewed the database from inception until 2020, included controlled studies of AS treated with NSAIDs or biologics and reports of CV events. The results showed that with NSAID use, no increased risk of CV events was observed and the risk of CVA was significantly reduced (RR of 0.58). TNF inhibitor (TNFi) use did not show an increased risk of MI, though specific data on CV events was limited.[61]

Additional population studies also supported the idea that NSAIDs in AS may be protective. A case-control study to investigate the risk of CVD following NSAID use in patients with AS used the Taiwanese claims database spanning from 1997 to 2008 where they identified 10,763 AS patients and 421 with CVD. When compared to age- and sex-matched controls, AS patients had increased risk of CVD (OR 1.68), frequent cyclooxygenase-II (COX-II) users had a ten times lower risk at 24 months, and frequent NSAID users had a significantly lower risk of MACE at 12 months (OR 0.23). However, non-frequent NSAID users and short-term exposure for less than 6 months did carry a higher risk, but this no longer existed after 12 months.[62] Other studies have also suggested the potential safety of COX-II inhibitors and various other effects of NSAIDs in AS patients.[63,64]

A Norwegian study also showed that one of the factors associated with an increased risk of reduced life expectancy was the lack of NSAID use (OR 4.53). Ogdie et al. reported that risk of MACE was higher in patients with PsA who were not using DMARDs.[65] In psoriasis, a retrospective study analyzed 7,000 American veterans who had been treated with methotrexate (MTX) for psoriasis and RA and found a significantly reduced incidence of CVD in these patients.[64]

BIOLOGICS

The effects of TNFis, MTX, NSAIDs, and corticosteroids on CV events in RA/psoriasis and PsA were the focus of a systematic review and meta-analysis covering articles from 1960 to 2012, including only six studies for PsO and PsA. The only conclusion that could be reached was that systemic therapy showed a significant decrease in risk of all CV events in PsO/PsA with an RR 0.75. From the RA patients, TNFis and MTX were associated with a reduction in risk, while NSAIDs and corticosteroids were associated with an increase in risk of all CV events.[66]

Using the Israeli health services data including 4,076 AS patients found that the proportion of IHD was higher among AS patients as compared to controls (14.1% vs 6.36%). Patients treated with anti-TNFs had a lower risk for IHD compared to non-anti-TNF users. However, after adjusting for risk factors of HTN, hyperlipidemia, DM, and smoking, AS was not found to be significantly associated with IHD and anti-TNF therapy was not found to be protective.[12] In a more recent study evaluating the use of DMARDs, it was found that treatment with conventional DMARDs was associated with a lower HR death, whereas treatment with biologic DMARDs was associated with a similar trend but was not statistically significant. Their conclusion suggested that a reduction in mortality with treatment optimization may be present, but this may be more difficult to achieve for those with severe disease (as defined by patients requiring biologic DMARDs).[42] In a 2020 systematic review and meta-analysis looking at the effect of therapies for AS and their effect on CV events were examined. Non-selective NSAID use was not associated with an increased risk of CVE, and in fact, risk for CVA was lower in NSAID users. There was also no significant association between TNFi and MI.[61]

In a population of PsA patients (120 on TNF blockers and 104 on DMARDs), a lower IMT at the common carotid and at the carotid bifurcation was noted in TNF-treated patients as compared with DMARD-treated patients (DiMinno et al. 2015). JAK inhibitor treatment for PsA (783) and psoriasis (3,663) with a median duration of 2–3 years with a coexistent metabolic syndrome in 40.9% and 32.7% showed an increased incidence of IRs for MACE especially in patients with a greater than 20% ASCVD 10-year risk.[19]

MONITORING FOR CVD IN SPONDYLOARTHROPATHY

In 2010 and updated in 2016, EULAR released ten recommendations regarding CVD management in patients with RA and other forms of inflammatory arthritis which included AS and PsA. The literature search spanned from 1966 to 2008 and then extended to 2015 and included 234 studies in RA, 17 in AS, and 13 in PsA. Their recommendations included that risk score models should be adapted for inflammatory arthritis and should use a 1.5 multiplication factor in RA, and this may be applicable to AS and PsA. They attributed this increased risk to both traditional risk factors and inflammatory burden. They recommended CVD risk assessment in all patients with RA, AS, or

PsA every 5 years or with any major changes in therapy. In addition, adequate control of disease activity was deemed necessary to lower CV risk. They also focused attention on the total cholesterol/high-density lipoprotein ratio. Patients with inflammatory arthritis and active disease tend to have low HDLs which causes the TC/HDL ratio to be high. This ratio is considered an important prognostic indicator for future CV risk. The recommendations also mention the preference for use of statins, ACE inhibitors, and angiotensin receptor blockers to treat comorbidities due to their potential anti-inflammatory effect. NSAIDs and corticosteroids are recommended to be used cautiously and at the lowest dose possible. Finally, one of the overarching principles is that the rheumatologist is responsible for CVD risk management in patients with RA and other inflammatory joint diseases.[68]

SUMMARY

While the increased risk of CVD and mortality appears consistent in studies of RA patients, the results concerning spondyloarthritis patients are more divergent. However, an increased risk of CVD is likely associated with AS and PsA though it is also clear that these populations also have increased prevalence of traditional CV risk factors. The data about increased CV risk is inconsistent in the literature and perhaps due to the bidirectional effects of NSAIDs and biologic DMARDs on CV risk. High disease activity and severity in AS, psoriasis, and PsA do seem to increase CV risk and mortality. However, the effect of decreasing inflammation with NSAIDs and biologics may not result in a significant decrease in CV mortality. In addition, though CVE risk is increased in the general population and RA patients using NSAIDs, the CVE risk in AS patients using NSAIDs is not clear. Several studies conclude that CV risk is underestimated in AS and PsA patients. This patient population would benefit from more careful screening, monitoring, and treatment of traditional CV risk factors.

REFERENCES

1. Rudwaleit M, et al. The development of Assessment of SpondyloArthritis international Society classification criteria for axial spondyloarthritis (part II): validation and final selection. Ann Rheum Dis. 2009;68:777–783.
2. Buleu F, et al. Heart involvement in inflammatory rheumatic disease: a systematic literature review. Medicina. 2019;55(6):249.
3. Nurmohamed MT, et al. Cardiovascular comorbidity in rheumatic diseases. Nat Rev Rheumatol. 2015;11(12):693–694.
4. Wolfe F, et al. The National Data Bank for rheumatic diseases: a multi-registry rheumatic disease data bank. Rheumatology. 2011;50(1):16–24.
5. Goodson N, et al. Cardiovascular admissions and mortality in an inception cohort of patients with rheumatoid arthritis with onset in the 1980's and 1990's. Ann Rheum Dis. 2005 Nov;64(11):1595–1601.
6. Han C, et al. Cardiovascular disease and risk factors in patients with rheumatoid arthritis, psoriatic arthritis and ankylosing spondylitis. J Rheumatol. 2006 Nov;33(11):2167–2172.
7. Bengtsson K, et al. Are ankylosing spondylitis, psoriatic arthritis and undifferentiated spondyloarthritis associated with an increased risk of cardiovascular events: a prospective nationwide population-based cohort study. Arthritis Res Ther. 2017;19(1):102.
8. Novelli I, et al. Extra-articular manifestations and comorbidities in psoriatic disease: a journey into the immunologic crosstalk. Front Med. 2021;8:737079.
9. Radford EP, et al. Mortality among patients with ankylosing spondylitis not given X-ray therapy. N Engl J Med. 1977;297:572–576.
10. Hollan I, et al. Spondyloarthritis: a strong predictor of early coronary artery bypass grafting. Scan J Rheumatol. 2008;37(1):18–22.
11. Huang JX, et al. Benefits of tumor necrosis factor inhibitors for cardiovascular disease in ankylosing spondylitis. Int Immunopharmacol. 2022;112:109207.
12. Shuster MV, et al. Ischemic heart disease and ankylosing spondylitis-assessing the role of inflammation. Clin Rheumatol. 2018;37(4):1053–1058.

13. Eriksson JK, et al. Is ankylosing spondylitis a risk factor for cardiovascular disease, and how do these risks compare with those in rheumatoid arthritis? Ann Rheum Dis. 2017;76:364.

14. Schieir O, et al. Incident myocardial infarction associated with major types of arthritis in the general population: a systemic review and meta-analysis. Ann Rheum Dis. 2017;76(8):1396–1404.

15. Mathieu S, et al. Cardiovascular events in ankylosing spondylitis: an updated meta-analysis. Semin Arthritis Rheum. 2015;44:551–555.

16. Ungprasert P, et al. Risk of coronary artery disease in patients with ankylosing spondylitis: a systematic review and meta-analysis. Ann Transl Med. 2015;3(4):51.

17. Sodergren A, et al. Characteristics and outcome of a first acute myocardial infarction in patients with ankylosing spondylitis. Clin Rheumatol. 2021;40(4):1321–1329.

18. Carter ET, et al. Epidemiology of ankylosing spondylitis in Rochester, Minnesota, 1935-1973. Arthritis Rheum. 1979;22(4):365–370.

19. Toussirot E. The risk of cardiovascular disease in axial spondyloarthritis. Current insights. Front Med. 2021;8:782150.

20. Lehitenen K. Mortality and causes of death in 398 patients admitted to hospital with ankylosing spondylitis. Ann Rheum Dis. 1993;52:174–176.

21. Bakland G, et al. Increased mortality in ankylosing spondylitis is related to disease activity. Ann Rheum Dis. 2011 Nov;70(11):1921–1925.

22. Exarchou S, et al. Mortality in ankylosing spondylitis: results from a nationwide population-based study. Ann Rheum Dis. 2016;75:1466–1472.

23. Haroon NN, et al. Patients with ankylosing spondylitis have increased cardiovascular and cerebrovascular mortality: a population-based study. Ann Intern Med. 2015;163:409.

24. Bergfeldt L. HLA-B27-associated cardiac disease. Ann Intern Med. 1997;127(8):621–629.

25. Forsblad-d'Elia H, et al. Cardiac conduction system abnormalities in ankylosing spondylitis: a cross-sectional study. BMC Musculoskelet Disord. 2013;14:237.

26. Roldan CA, et al. Aortic root disease and valve disease associated with ankylosing spondylitis. J Am Coll Cardiol. 1998;32:1397–1402.

27. Bengtsson K, et al. Risk of cardiac rhythm disturbances and aortic regurgitation in different spondyloarthritis subtypes in comparison with general population: a register-based study from Sweden. Ann Rheum Dis. 2018;77(4):541–548.

28. Bengtsson K, et al. Cardiac conduction disturbances in patients with ankylosing spondylitis: results from a 5-year follow-up cohort study. RMD Open. 2019;5(2):e001053.

29. Szabo SM, et al. Increased risk of cardiovascular and cerebrovascular diseases in individuals with ankylosing spondylitis: a population-based study. Arthritis Rheum. 2011;63(11):3294–3304.

30. Moon I, et al. Ankylosing spondylitis: a novel risk factor for atrial fibrillation – a nationwide population-based study. Int J Cardiol. 2019;275:77–82.

31. Baniaamam M, et al. The prevalence of cardiac diseases in a contemporary large cohort of Dutch elderly ankylosing spondylitis patients – the CARDAS study. J Clin Med. 2021;10:5069.

32. Brunner F, et al. Ankylosing spondylitis and heart abnormalities: do cardiac conduction disorders, valve regurgitation and diastolic dysfunction occur more often in male patients diagnosed with ankylosing spondylitis for over 15 years than in the normal population. Clin Rheumatol. 2006;25:24.

33. Morovatdar N, et al. Ankylosing spondylitis and risk of cardiac arrhythmia and conduction disorders: a systematic review and meta-analysis. Curr Cardiol Rev. 2021;17(5):e150521193326.

34. Mease PH, et al. Characterization of patients with ankylosing spondylitis and nonradiographic axial spondyloarthritis in the US-based corrona registry. Arthritis Care Res. 2018;70(11):1661–1670.

35. Zhao SS, et al. Comparison of comorbidities and treatment between ankylosing spondylitis and non-radiographic axial spondyloarthritis in the United States. Rheumatology. 2019;58(11):2025–2030.

36. Villani AP, et al. Prevalence of undiagnosed psoriatic arthritis among psoriasis patients: systematic review and meta-analysis. J Am Acad Dermatol. 2015;73:242.

37. Scarpa R, et al. Psoriasis, psoriatic arthritis or psoriatic disease? J Rheumatol. 2006;33(2):210–212.

38. Gupta S, et al. Comorbidities in psoriatic arthritis: a systematic review and meta-analysis. Rheumatol Int. 2021;41:275–284.

39. Ali Y, et al. Improved survival in psoriatic arthritis with calendar time. Arthritis Rheum. 2007;56(8):2708–2714.

40. Mok CC, et al. Life expectancy, standardized mortality ratios, and causes of death in six rheumatic diseases in Hong Kong, China. Arthritis Rheum. 2011;63(5):1182–1189.

41. Leung YY. Is psoriatic arthritis associated with higher risk of mortality? J Rheumatol. 2022 Feb;49(2):128–131.

42. Haddad A, et al. The association of psoriatic arthritis with all-cause mortality and leading causes of death in psoriatic arthritis. J Rheumatol. 2022 Feb;49(2):165–170.

43. Ahlehoff O, et al. Psoriasis is associated with clinically significant cardiovascular risk: a Danish nationwide cohort study. J Intern Med. 2011;270(2):147–157.

44. Armstrong AW, et al. Psoriasis prevalence in adults in the United States. JAMA Dermatol. 2021;157(8):940–946.

45. Gelfand JM, et al. Risk of myocardial infarction in patients with psoriasis. JAMA. 2006;296:1735–1741.

46. Kaye JA, Li L, Jack SS. Incidence of risk factors for myocardial infarction and other vascular disease in patients with psoriasis. Br J Dermatol. 2008;159:895–902.

47. Brauchli YB, et al. Psoriasis and risk of ancient myocardial infarction, stroke or transient ischaemic attack: an inception cohort study with a nested case-control analysis. Br J Dermal. 2009;160(5):1048–1056.

48. Mallbris L, et al. Increased risk for cardiovascular mortality in psoriasis inpatients but not in outpatients. Eur J Epidemiol. 2004;19:225–230.

49. Rueda-Gotor J, et al. Cardiovascular and disease-related features associated with extra-articular manifestations in axial spondyloarthritis. A multi-center study of 888 patients. Semin Arthritis Rheum. 2022;57:152096.

50. Miller I, et al. Quantifying cardiovascular disease risk factors in patients with psoriasis: a meta-analysis. Br J Dermal. 2013;169:1180–1187.

51. Tobin AM, et al. Cardiovascular disease and risk factors in patients with psoriasis and psoriatic arthritis. J Rheumatol. 2010;37(7):1386–1394.

52. Lai Y-F, et al. Uveitis as a risk factor for developing acute myocardial infarction in ankylosing spondylitis: a national population-based longitudinal cohort study. Front Immune. 2022;12:811664.

53. Berg IJ, et al. Uveitis is associated with hypertension and atherosclerosis in patients with ankylosing spondylitis: a cross-sectional study. Semin Arthritis Rheum. 2014;44(3):309–313.

54. Gao X, et al. Association between atherosclerosis-related cardiovascular disease and uveitis: a systematic review and meta-analysis. Diagnostics. 2022;12(12):3178.

55. Biondi RB, et al. Cardiovascular risk in individuals with inflammatory bowel disease. Coin Exp Gastroenterol. 2020;13:107–113.

56. Rungoe C, et al. Risk of ischemic heart disease in patients with inflammatory bowel disease: a nationwide Danish cohort study. Gut. 2013;62:689–694.

57. Kristensen SL, et al. Disease activity in inflammatory bowel disease is associated with increased risk of myocardial infarction, stroke and cardiovascular death—a Danish nationwide cohort study. PLOS ONE. 2013;8(2):e56944.

58. Feng KM, et al. Increased risk of acute coronary syndrome in ankylosing spondylitis patients with uveitis: a population-based cohort study. Front Immune. 2022;13:890543.

59. Tam HW, et al. Sulfasalzine might reduce risk of cardiovascular diseases in patients with ankylosing spondylitis: a nationwide population-based retrospective cohort study. Int J Rheum Dis. 2017;20:363–370.

60. Oza A, et al. Survival benefit of statin use in ankylosing spondylitis: a general population-based cohort study. Ann Rheum Dis. 2017;76(10):1737–1742.

61. Karmacharya P, et al. Effects of therapies on cardiovascular events in ankylosing spondylitis: a systematic review and meta-analysis. Rheumatol Ther. 2020;7(4):993–1009.

62. Tsai WC, et al. Long-term frequent use of non-steroidal anti-inflammatory drugs might protect patients with ankylosing spondylitis from cardiovascular diseases: a nationwide case-control study. PLOS ONE. 2015;10(5):e0126347.

63. Nissen SE, et al. Cardiovascular safety of celecoxib, naproxen, or ibuprofen for arthritis. N Engl J Med. 2016;375:2519–2529.

64. Liew JW, et al. Cardiovascular morbidity and mortality in ankylosing spondylitis and psoriatic arthritis. Best Pract Clip Rheumatol. 2018;32(3):369–389.

65. Prodanovich S, et al. Methotrexate reduces incidence of vascular diseases in veterans with psoriasis or rheumatoid arthritis. J Am Acad Dermal. 2005;52:262.

66. Ogdie A, et al. Risk of major cardiovascular events in patients with psoriatic arthritis, psoriasis and rheumatoid arthritis: a population-based cohort study. Ann Rheum Dis. 2015;74(2):326.

67. Di Minno MN, et al. Carotid intima-media thickness in psoriatic arthritis: differences between tumor necrosis factor-α blockers and traditional disease-modifying antirheumatic drugs. Arteriosclerosis, thrombosis, and vascular biology. 2011 Mar;31(3):705–712.

68. Agca R, et al. EULAR recommendations for cardiovascular disease risk management in patients with rheumatoid arthritis and other forms of inflammatory joint disorders: 2015/2016 update. Ann Rheum Dis. 2016;76(1):17–28.

5

Gout and hyperuricemia in cardiovascular disease

CHRISTOPHER HINO, DANA SONG, AND SOPHIA LI

INTRODUCTION

Gout represents one of the most common inflammatory arthropathies worldwide, affecting approximately 4% of adults (9.2 million people) per year in the United States.[1] The deposition of monosodium urate (MSU) in peripheral joints and surrounding tissues leads to acute articular and periarticular inflammation, resulting in intense and painful arthritis during acute episodes. Although these episodes are often self-limited, the overall disease contributes to substantial morbidity. Moreover, emerging evidence suggests that systemic inflammation from gout can increase the risk of cardiovascular disease.

PATHOPHYSIOLOGY

Uric acid (UA) is the final metabolic product of purine metabolism. In humans, UA can be derived exogenously from purine-containing diets (especially in alcohol, meat, or seafood) or endogenously produced in the liver, intestines, muscles, kidneys, and vascular endothelium.[2] The two purine nucleic acids, adenine and guanine, are degraded in the liver through a series of complex metabolic pathways that converge to produce hypoxanthine, which is then oxidized by xanthine dehydrogenase to produce xanthine and then UA (Figure 5.1).[3] Unlike most mammals, humans and some non-human primates are unable to oxidize UA to the more soluble allantoin due to the absence of uricase enzyme.[4] Consequently, humans and several other primates have higher levels of UA, which must be excreted through the kidney (65–75%) and intestinal tract (25–35%). Serum UA levels normally range between 1.5 and 6.0 mg/dL in women and 2.5 and 7.0 mg/dL in men. Under physiologic conditions, UA exists as a weak acid in its deprotonated ionic form. However, when UA levels are higher than 7 mg/dL, UA crystallizes to form MSU. The urate crystals can then deposit into soft tissues and joints, inciting an acute, inflammatory response through Toll-like receptor 2 (TLR2)/Toll-like receptor 4 (TLR4) and NOD-like receptor protein 3 (NLRP3) inflammasome activation, resulting in pain, erythema, and swelling.[5]

Elevated levels of UA have also been associated with diseases, such as hypertension, diabetes, atherosclerosis, chronic kidney disease, and atrial fibrillation (AF), suggesting that it may also have deleterious effects depending on the chemical microenvironment.[6–9] While the exact mechanism by which UA may promote disease remains to be fully elucidated, experimental studies have shown that hyperuricemia is associated with endothelial dysfunction, intracellular oxidative stress, and renin–angiotensin–aldosterone system activation in humans.[10,11] For example, studies have shown that radical oxygen species produced during the oxidation of xanthine and

DOI: 10.1201/9781003386711-5

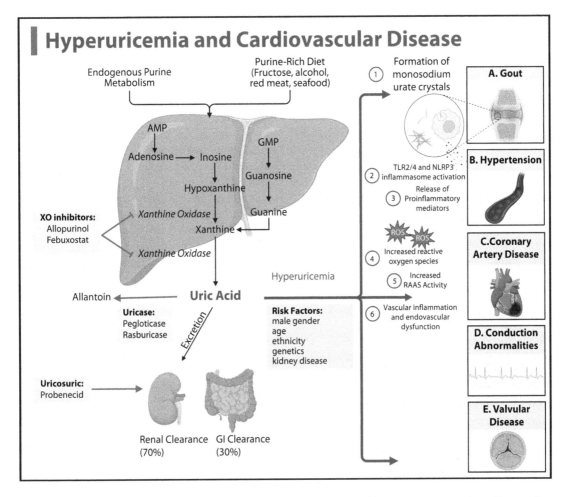

Figure 5.1 Graphic illustration of the proposed pathophysiology of hyperuricemia and cardiovascular disease. Elements of the figure were created in Biorender.com.

hypoxanthine by xanthine oxidase may damage endothelial cells.[12] There is also evidence that UA may also directly induce inflammation in endothelial cells and proliferation of vascular smooth muscle cells through increased MCP-1 expression and activation of NF-kB, MAPK, and COX-2 pathways.[13,14]

CARDIOVASCULAR DISEASE MANIFESTATIONS

Associations between gout and cardiovascular disease have been well studied, though the causal relationship remains an area of active investigation. Here we review current evidence of cardiovascular disease manifestations in gout.

Hypertension

Hypertension (HTN) is one of the most common comorbidities associated with gout. Based on the US National Health and Nutrition Examination Survey, an estimated 74% of patients with gout also have hypertension.[15] Similarly, approximately 25% of patients with untreated hypertension and 75% of patients with malignant hypertension are found to have hyperuricemia.[16] These findings have been further supported in multiple large epidemiological studies showing hyperuricemia is a strong independent predictor of hypertension, even when controlling for age, gender, race, and cholesterol level.[17,18]

Several preclinical studies have attempted to establish hyperuricemia as a causality for hypertension.

For example, researchers have found that direct injection of UA into rabbits or induction of mild hyperuricemia using oxonic acid (a uricase inhibitor) in rodents have been shown to induce hypertension in a dose dependent manner.[19,20] Importantly, the development of hypertension was prevented by concurrent treatment with UA-lowering therapies, such as allopurinol, a xanthine oxidase inhibitor, or benziodarone, a uricosuric agent.[20]

Based on these observations, UA-lowering therapies have been suggested as one possible therapeutic approach to managing hypertension. In this regard, several randomized controlled trials have investigated the efficacy of UA-lowering therapies on blood pressure (BP). In one randomized, double-blind, placebo-controlled, crossover trial, researchers evaluated the impact of urate-lowering therapy on 30 adolescents aged 11–17 years with newly diagnosed hypertension and UA levels >6 mg/dL. The mean change in systolic BP was approximately 6.9 mmHg (95% confidence interval [CI]: −4.5 to 9.3 mmHg) in the treatment group (allopurinol 200 mg twice daily for 4 weeks) compared to −2.0 mmHg (95% CI, 0.3 to −4.3 mmHg; P=0.009) in the placebo group. Importantly, they found that 20 of the 30 participants achieved normal BP while taking allopurinol, compared to 1 participant while taking placebo (P<0.001).[21]

Another randomized, double-blind, placebo-controlled trial compared the use of either allopurinol, probenecid, or placebo in 60 prehypertensive, obese adolescent children aged 11–17 years. After 2 months of treatment, patients who had received urate-lowering therapy were found to have a decrease in systolic BP of approximately 10.2 mmHg, compared to a rise of 1.7 mmHg in the placebo group.[22]

Coronary artery disease and myocardial infarction

Coronary artery disease (CAD), the most common type of heart disease in the United States, affects approximately 20 million adults aged 20 years and older.[23] Gout has been linked to hyperlipidemia and obesity. As such, the relationship between gout and CAD has been studied. In one retrospective study following patients undergoing cardiac catheterization

with obstructive CAD, gout diagnosis at the time of catheterization was shown to worsen all-cause mortality (hazard ratio [HR]: 1.13, 95% CI: 1.05–1.23; P=0.002) in patients with preexisting CAD.[24] While the etiology is not confirmed, the oxidative stress and inflammation in gout are theorized to potentially play an important role. Interestingly, the patients in the study were already on optimal medical therapy for cardiovascular disease. Therefore, it is crucial to investigate whether gout medications can bridge this gap and help prevent adverse outcomes in patients with CAD and gout. A randomized controlled crossover trial studied the impact of allopurinol use on exercise tolerance testing in patients with stable chronic angina. The study demonstrated that, when compared to placebo, the completion of a 6-week allopurinol course prolonged the median time to ECG changes of ST segment depression, total exercise time, and time to angina during exercise tolerance testing.[25] Given that the majority of myocardial infarctions (MIs) are secondary to CAD, it is not surprising that gout and hyperuricemia were also demonstrated to be independent risk factors for MI in several studies.[26–28] Other studies have shown that allopurinol use is associated with a decreased risk of MI.[29–31]

Conduction abnormalities

Gout has also demonstrated an association with an increased risk of developing AF.[32,33] A study using US Medicare data from 2005 to 2012 demonstrated that a gout diagnosis almost doubled the risk of AF incidence in the elderly.[34] The underlying etiology is unclear, though studies have demonstrated that inflammatory markers such as interleukin (IL)-6 and C-reactive protein play a role in the development of AF. As such, it is theorized that the systemic inflammation in gout may contribute to the increased risk of AF.[32,33] In line with gouty association with AF, several studies have shown a direct correlation between increased serum UA levels and AF.[35,36] Interestingly, prophylactic colchicine has demonstrated its ability to reduce the incidence of AF after cardiac surgery or intervention in several randomized controlled trials.[37] Together, these studies suggest that treating hyperuricemia and inflammation in gout may help prevent AF.

Valvular disease

The relationship between gout and valvular disease has not been well established, although there has been emerging research investigating the association of aortic stenosis and gout. A retrospective study demonstrated that patients with aortic stenosis had an increased likelihood of being diagnosed with gout compared to patients without aortic stenosis (adjusted odds ratio 2.08, 95% CI 1.00–4.32; P=0.049).[38] The same research group published a second retrospective study, which showed that in a patient population with aortic stenosis, those with an additional diagnosis of gout had an increased likelihood of progressing to severe aortic stenosis when compared to those without gout (74% vs 54%; P=0.001; HR 1.45, 95% CI 1.09–1.93).[39] The exact mechanism is unclear, though there have been case reports regarding valvular tophi depositions leading to valvular diseases involving the aortic valve, as well as the mitral valve and pulmonary valve.[40–42] While this is a rare phenomenon, valvular tophi should be on the differential in patients with gout who otherwise do not show symptoms of infective endocarditis but have cardiac echocardiogram findings suggestive of vegetations.

THERAPEUTIC MANAGEMENT

Urate-lowering therapies have been instrumental in the management of gout. These treatments include allopurinol and febuxostat, which are xanthine oxidase inhibitors that prevent the conversion of hypoxanthine and xanthine to UA, probenecid, an organic anion transporter inhibitor that prevents reabsorption of UA in the renal tubules, and pegloticase, a uricase that converts UA to allantoin. As discussed above, there have been studies that have shown how urate-lowering therapies may help manage or prevent cardiovascular diseases such as hypertension and AF. Of note, there was initial concern for an increased risk of cardiovascular deaths with the use of febuxostat when compared to allopurinol based on the Cardiovascular Safety of Febuxostat or Allopurinol in Patients with Gout (CARES) trial published in 2018.[43] This study led to a febuxostat black box warning that it may increase the risk of cardiovascular deaths in those with underlying cardiovascular disease. Subsequent studies, including the long-term cardiovascular safety of febuxostat compared with allopurinol in patients with gout (FAST) trial, did not confirm this association and instead found no relationship between febuxostat and an increased risk of cardiovascular death.[44] Moreover, discontinuing febuxostat or allopurinol in patients with gout was linked to an increased risk of cardiovascular death in a separate study.[45]

CONCLUDING REMARKS

A large body of evidence has demonstrated a close association among gout, hyperuricemia, and the risk for cardiovascular disease, including hypertension, MI, AF, and valvular disease. The role of urate-lowering treatments in improving cardiovascular outcomes remains an area of ongoing research, though current evidence does suggest that treating the underlying inflammation and hyperuricemia in gout may lead to improved cardiovascular outcomes. Further investigation uncovering the relationship between gout and cardiovascular disease will be necessary to develop new prevention and treatment strategies.

REFERENCES

1. Chen-Xu M, Yokose C, Rai SK, Pillinger MH, Choi HK. Contemporary prevalence of gout and hyperuricemia in the United States and decadal trends: the National Health and Nutrition Examination Survey, 2007–2016. Arthritis Rheumatol Hoboken NJ. 2019 Jun;71(6):991–999.
2. Chaudhary K, Malhotra K, Sowers J, Aroor A. Uric acid – key ingredient in the recipe for cardiorenal metabolic syndrome. Cardiorenal Med. 2013 Oct;3(3):208–220.
3. Maiuolo J, Oppedisano F, Gratteri S, Muscoli C, Mollace V. Regulation of uric acid metabolism and excretion. Int J Cardiol. 2016 Jun 15;213:8–14.
4. Wu XW, Muzny DM, Lee CC, Caskey CT. Two independent mutational events in the loss of urate oxidase during hominoid evolution. J Mol Evol. 1992 Jan;34(1):78–84.
5. Dalbeth N, Gosling AL, Gaffo A, Abhishek A. Gout. Lancet. 2021 May 15;397(10287):1843–1855.
6. Kuwabara M, Borghi C, Cicero AFG, Hisatome I, Niwa K, Ohno M, et al. Elevated serum uric acid increases risks

for developing high LDL cholesterol and hypertriglyceridemia: a five-year cohort study in Japan. Int J Cardiol. 2018 Jun 15;261:183–188.

7. Kuwabara M, Kuwabara R, Hisatome I, Niwa K, Roncal-Jimenez CA, Bjornstad P, et al. "Metabolically healthy" obesity and hyperuricemia increase risk for hypertension and diabetes: 5-year Japanese cohort study. Obesity. 2017;25(11):1997–2008.

8. Kuwabara M, Niwa K, Nishihara S, Nishi Y, Takahashi O, Kario K, et al. Hyperuricemia is an independent competing risk factor for atrial fibrillation. Int J Cardiol. 2017 Mar 15;231:137–142.

9. Morikawa N, Bancks MP, Yano Y, Kuwabara M, Gaffo AL, Duprez DA, et al. Serum urate trajectory in young adulthood and incident cardiovascular disease events by middle age: CARDIA study. Hypertension. 2021 Nov;78(5):1211–1218.

10. Milanesi S, Verzola D, Cappadona F, Bonino B, Murugavel A, Pontremoli R, et al. Uric acid and angiotensin II additively promote inflammation and oxidative stress in human proximal tubule cells by activation of toll-like receptor 4. J Cell Physiol. 2019 Jul;234(7):10868–10876.

11. Yu W, Cheng JD. Uric acid and cardiovascular disease: an update from molecular mechanism to clinical perspective. Front Pharmacol [Internet]. 2020;11. Available from: https://www.frontiersin.org/articles/10.3389/fphar.2020.582680

12. McCord JM. Oxygen-derived free radicals in postischemic tissue injury. N Engl J Med. 1985 Jan 17;312(3):159–163.

13. Kimura Y, Tsukui D, Kono H. Uric acid in inflammation and the pathogenesis of atherosclerosis. Int J Mol Sci. 2021 Nov 17;22(22):12394.

14. Spiga R, Marini MA, Mancuso E, Di Fatta C, Fuoco A, Perticone F, et al. Uric acid is associated with inflammatory biomarkers and induces inflammation via activating the NF-κB signaling pathway in HepG2 cells. Arterioscler Thromb Vasc Biol. 2017 Jun;37(6):1241–1249.

15. Zhu Y, Pandya BJ, Choi HK. Prevalence of gout and hyperuricemia in the US general population: the National Health and Nutrition Examination Survey 2007-2008. Arthritis Rheum. 2011 Oct;63(10):3136–3141.

16. Cannon PJ, Stason WB, Demartini FE, Sommers SC, Laragh JH. Hyperuricemia in primary and renal hypertension. N Engl J Med. 1966 Sep 1;275(9):457–464.

17. Borghi C, Agnoletti D, Cicero AFG, Lurbe E, Virdis A. Uric acid and hypertension: a review of evidence and future perspectives for the management of cardiovascular risk. Hypertension. 2022 Sep;79(9):1927–1936.

18. Stewart DJ, Langlois V, Noone D. Hyperuricemia and hypertension: links and risks. Integr Blood Press Control. 2019 Dec 24;12:43–62.

19. Desgrez A. Influence de la constitution des corps puriques sure leur action vis-a-vis de la pression arterielle. Comptes Rendus L'Academie Sci. 1913;156:93–94.

20. Mazzali M, Hughes J, Kim YG, Jefferson JA, Kang DH, Gordon KL, et al. Elevated uric acid increases blood pressure in the rat by a novel crystal-independent mechanism. Hypertension. 2001 Nov;38(5):1101–1106.

21. Feig DI, Soletsky B, Johnson RJ. Effect of allopurinol on blood pressure of adolescents with newly diagnosed essential hypertension: a randomized trial. JAMA J Am Med Assoc. 2008 Aug 27;300(8):924–932.

22. Soletsky B, Feig DI. Uric acid reduction rectifies prehypertension in obese adolescents. Hypertension. 2012 Nov;60(5):1148–1156.

23. CDC. Heart Disease Facts [Internet]. Centers for Diseases Control and Prevention. Available from: https://www.cdc.gov/heartdisease/facts.htm. Accessed 20 February 2024.

24. Pagidipati NJ, Clare RM, Keenan RT, Chiswell K, Roe MT, Hess CN. Association of gout with long-term cardiovascular outcomes among patients with obstructive coronary artery disease. J Am Heart Assoc. 2018 Aug 21;7(16):e009328.

25. Noman A, Ang DS, Ogston S, Lang CC, Struthers AD. Effect of high-dose allopurinol on exercise in patients with chronic

stable angina: a randomised, placebo controlled crossover trial. Lancet. 2010 Jun 19;375(9732):2161–2167.

26. Singh JA, Cleveland JD. Gout and the risk of myocardial infarction in older adults: a study of Medicare recipients. Arthritis Res Ther. 2018 Jun 1;20(1):109.

27. Krishnan E, Baker JF, Furst DE, Schumacher HR. Gout and the risk of acute myocardial infarction. Arthritis Rheum. 2006 Aug;54(8):2688–2696.

28. Liu SC, Xia L, Zhang J, Lu XH, Hu DK, Zhang HT, et al. Gout and risk of myocardial infarction: a systematic review and meta-analysis of cohort studies. PLOS ONE. 2015 Jul 31;10(7):e0134088.

29. Singh JA, Yu S. Allopurinol reduces the risk of myocardial infarction (MI) in the elderly: a study of medicare claims. Arthritis Res Ther. 2016 Sep 22;18(1):209.

30. de Abajo FJ, Gil MJ, Rodríguez A, García-Poza P, Álvarez A, Bryant V, et al. Allopurinol use and risk of non-fatal acute myocardial infarction. Heart. 2015 May 1;101(9):679–685.

31. Grimaldi-Bensouda L, Alpérovitch A, Aubrun E, Danchin N, Rossignol M, Abenhaim L, et al. Impact of allopurinol on risk of myocardial infarction. Ann Rheum Dis. 2015 May 1;74(5):836–842.

32. Kim SC, Liu J, Solomon DH. Risk of incident atrial fibrillation in gout: a cohort study. Ann Rheum Dis. 2016 Aug 1;75(8):1473–1478.

33. Kuo CF, Grainge MJ, Mallen C, Zhang W, Doherty M. Impact of gout on the risk of atrial fibrillation. Rheumatology. 2016 Apr 1;55(4):721–728.

34. Singh JA, Cleveland JD. Gout and the risk of incident atrial fibrillation in older adults: a study of US Medicare data. RMD Open. 2018 Jul 13;4(2):e000712.

35. Kawasoe S, Kubozono T, Yoshifuku S, Ojima S, Oketani N, Miyata M, et al. Uric acid level and prevalence of atrial fibrillation in a Japanese general population of 285,882. Circ J Off J Jpn Circ Soc. 2016 Nov 25;80(12):2453–2459.

36. Tamariz L, Hernandez F, Bush A, Palacio A, Hare JM. Association between serum uric acid and atrial fibrillation: a systematic review and meta-analysis. Heart Rhythm. 2014 Jul;11(7):1102–1108.

37. Zhao H, Chen Y, Mao M, Yang J, Chang J. A meta-analysis of colchicine in prevention of atrial fibrillation following cardiothoracic surgery or cardiac intervention. J Cardiothorac Surg. 2022 Sep 1;17:224.

38. Chang K, Yokose C, Tenner C, Oh C, Donnino R, Choy-Shan A, et al. Association between gout and aortic stenosis. Am J Med. 2017 Feb;130(2):230.e1–230.e8.

39. Adelsheimer A, Shah B, Choy-Shan A, Tenner CT, Lorin JD, Smilowitz NR, et al. Gout and progression of aortic stenosis. Am J Med. 2020 Sep;133(9):1095–1100.e1.

40. LaMoreaux B, Chandrasekaran V. Ab0876 gout causing urate cardiac vegetations: summary of published cases. Ann Rheum Dis. 2019 Jun 1;78(Suppl 2):1906–1906.

41. Scalapino JN, Edwards WD, Steckelberg JM, Wooten RS, Callahan JA, Ginsburg WW. Mitral stenosis associated with valvular tophi. Mayo Clin Proc. 1984 Jul;59(7):509–512.

42. Curtiss EI, Miller TR, Shapiro LS. Pulmonic regurgitation due to valvular tophi. Circulation. 1983 Mar;67(3):699–701.

43. White WB, Saag KG, Becker MA, Borer JS, Gorelick PB, Whelton A, et al. Cardiovascular safety of febuxostat or allopurinol in patients with gout. N Engl J Med. 2018 Mar 29;378(13):1200–1210.

44. Mackenzie IS, Ford I, Nuki G, Hallas J, Hawkey CJ, Webster J, et al. Long-term cardiovascular safety of febuxostat compared with allopurinol in patients with gout (FAST): a multicentre, prospective, randomised, open-label, non-inferiority trial. Lancet. 2020 Nov 28;396(10264):1745–1757.

45. Ghang BZ, Lee JS, Choi J, Kim J, Yoo B. Increased risk of cardiovascular events and death in the initial phase after discontinuation of febuxostat or allopurinol: another story of the CARES trial. RMD Open. 2022 Jun 1;8(2):e001944.

6

Osteoarthritis and cardiovascular disease: An evolving relationship

KARINA D. TORRALBA, ALPHA SHANIKA GONZALEZ,
AND C. KENT KWOH

INTRODUCTION

Osteoarthritis (OA) is a debilitating disease that affects all aspects of life.[1] Initially attributed to wear and tear, we now understand that OA is not only a condition involving structural damage to joint tissues, but also an illness, marked by an individual's experience of OA, with pain being the predominant symptom. Magnetic resonance imaging has provided evidence that OA is a heterogenous disease of the entire joint, causing structural damage to joint tissues.[2–4] It may involve all the joint tissues, including bone marrow lesions in the subchondral bone, synovitis, inflammation of Hoffa's fat pad, cartilage damage leading to denuded bone, osteophytes, meniscal extrusion, meniscal tear/maceration, and changes in trabecular bone texture in the subchondral bone. OA is the leading cause of pain and loss of function.[3–5] OA not only affects physical health, causing limitations in performing activities of daily living and decreased mobility, but also takes a toll on mental health. A study by the OA Initiative revealed that individuals with lower limb OA are at a greater risk for developing depressive symptoms and experiencing suicidal ideations compared to those without OA.[6]

Epidemiology

OA is one of the most common chronic joint diseases, affecting at least 240 million adults worldwide.[1] In 2012, the proportion of the population aged 45 and older with physician-diagnosed OA was 26.6%, and it is estimated to increase to 29.5% by 2032 globally.[7] The knees, hips, and hands are the most commonly affected by OA.[8] The prevalence of OA varies significantly based on the specific joint affected, with knee OA being the most studied form, constituting approximately 83% of all cases.[9] According to the National Health Interview Survey, an estimated 14 million people in the US have knee OA.[6]

Individuals with OA are at a 20% higher risk of comorbidities, including stroke and metabolic syndrome, compared to those without OA.[10] Up to 67% of individuals with OA have at least one other chronic condition, with stroke, peptic ulcer, and metabolic syndrome being the most common comorbidities.

Risk factors

OA can be classified as primary or secondary. Primary OA is the most common form and is diagnosed in the absence of trauma.[11] The pathogenesis

DOI: 10.1201/9781003386711-6

is poorly understood, but several risk factors are believed to play an important role in its incidence, including increasing age, obesity (BMI >30 kg/m), female gender, genetic predisposition, and joint injury or overuse.[5]

While aging is a risk factor, only approximately 50% of people develop OA in their lifetime.[12] Age contributes to OA through accumulation of unrepaired damaged DNA, telomere shortening, and the loss of tissue and organ function.[5] Obesity or a higher body weight significantly increased joint contact and adds stress to weight-bearing joints. Fat tissue can also lead to low levels of systemic inflammation.[5] Metabolic diseases, including diabetes mellitus (DM), can also increase the risk of hand OA.[13]

Women, compared to men, are more likely to develop hand, foot, and knee OA but are less likely to develop cervical spine OA.[6] Women aged 50–60 years old may be 350% more likely to develop hand OA as opposed to men in the same age range.[14] Women tend to report more severe OA than men.[14]

Approximately 39–78% of OA is attributable to genetic factors.[5] African Americans are more likely to develop symptomatic knee and hip OA.[6] Secondary OA is associated with a preexisting joint abnormality, such as trauma or disease.[11] The development and progression of secondary OA may or may not be influenced by the presence of the aforementioned risk factors. Post-traumatic arthritis, responsible for approximately 12% of all cases of OA, can occur at any age but is most commonly seen in younger adults. This type of arthritis develops after an episode of acute direct trauma to the joint.[15] Studies indicate that between 20% and more than 50% of patients may develop OA after joint trauma.[15]

Manifestations

There is currently no "gold standard" to aid reaching a diagnosis of OA. OA is a difficult disease to define as it has a variety of different clinical presentations. Diagnosis relies on typical clinical features and can be confirmed by plain radiographs. Classification criteria developed by the American College of Rheumatology are established to define homogenous subgroups for clinical studies and clinical trials. These criteria aid in distinguishing OA from more inflammatory disease such as rheumatoid arthritis.[16] Radiologic features of OA include osteophytes, narrowed joint spaces, subchondral bone thickening, and cysts on plain radiographs, as well as degradation of articular cartilage on MRI.[2,5] The widely used Kellgren and Lawrence grading system categorizes the severity of OA on a five-grade scale, ranging from Grade 0 (definite absence of X-ray changes of OA) to Grade 4 (severe OA).[9]

Typical symptoms of OA include pain exacerbated by physical activity, less than 30 minutes of morning stiffness, gelling, loss of mobility, feelings of joint insecurity or instability, and functional limitations.[17] A physical examination may reveal tender spots along the joint margins, firm bony swelling of the joint margin, crepitus, mild signs of inflammation (such as cool synovial effusions), restricted and painful range of motion, and joint instability. Large bony enlargement of joints may be manifested as Heberden's nodes on distal interphalangeal joints and Bouchard's nodes on the proximal interphalangeal joints, resulting from bone and cartilage remodeling.

Management

The goal of treatment is to alleviate pain and improve joint function, with the approach tailored to the stage and severity of disease. While imaging modalities are not mandatory to make a diagnosis, it is helpful to help determine and confirm structural damages.[7] A multi-disciplinary management plan is recommended, starting with education and non-pharmacological interventions for mild symptoms early in the disease course. As symptoms progress, and the disease becomes more severe, pharmacological options can be introduced.[18]

Pharmacologic therapies include nonselective nonsteroidal anti-inflammatory drugs (NSAIDs), selective cyclooxygenase-2 (COX-2) inhibitors, acetaminophen, tramadol, duloxetine, and intraarticular injections of corticosteroids.[8] Non-pharmacologic interventions include lifestyle modifications such as weight loss, assistive devices such as crutches and canes, acupuncture, heat/therapeutic cooling, kinesio taping, balance training, tai chi, exercise, and physical therapy.

Cardiovascular disease and OA

Cardiovascular diseases (CVDs) are leading causes of mortality worldwide, affecting approximately 17.3 million people.[19] CVD encompasses conditions such as coronary disease, including myocardial infarction (MI), ischemic heart disease (IHD), and congestive heart failure (CHF); cerebrovascular disease, including stroke and transient ischemic attack (TIA); peripheral arterial disease; rheumatic heart disease; congenital heart disease; deep venous thrombosis; and pulmonary embolism. Behavioral risk factors associated with the development of CVD include an unhealthy diet, sedentary lifestyle, and tobacco and alcohol use, leading to the development of hypercholesterolemia, hypertension, DM, and obesity. IHD, stroke, and TIA are more prevalent in populations above 50 years of age.

Common risk factors for OA and CVD

A number of studies have looked at the relationship between OA and CVD. Aging and obesity are common risk factors for both conditions (Table 6.1). Reducing obesity can be achieved through a combination of dietary alterations and increasing physical activity, which are key to treating both OA and CVD.[8,20–22] Central obesity is associated with the development of pain in OA. Obesity helps predict CVD and plays a role in CVD development in women with OA.[23]

Table 6.1 Distinguishing and shared risk factors of osteoarthritis and cardiovascular disease

	OA	CVD
Risk factors	Female gender	Hypertension
	Genetic predisposition	Hyperlipidemia
	Joint injury/ overuse	Diabetes
		Smoking/ secondhand smoke
	Age	
	Obesity	

Note: OA, Osteoarthritis; CVD, cardiovascular disease.

What do the studies tell us about the risk of CVD in OA?

A number of meta-analyses have studied the risk of CVD among patients with OA.[24] A significantly higher risk of MI and stroke was noted in 3550 OA subjects when compared to 2444 control subjects without OA.[25] Risk factors such as pro-atherogenic lipid profiles, high fasting glucose, and body mass index were identified. Metabolic syndrome and increased pulse wave velocities were higher in OA subjects. CVD was significantly elevated among 80,911 OA patients by 24% when compared with the general population of 29,213 patients (RR: 1.24, 95% CI: 1.12–1.37, P<0.001).[26] Interestingly, in a study that categorized OA according to weight-bearing status, an association with CVD was noted only for weight-bearing joints, while subclinical atherosclerosis was noted for all other OA affected joints.[27]

Not all manifestations of CVD may be associated with OA. When comparing OA cohorts with non-OA cohorts and their risk for CVD, the correlation varied: There was a three-fold decrease in TIA and an increased risk of CHF and IHD in OA cohorts, with no difference in MI or stroke between the two cohorts. The level of disability due to OA may also be a factor. While a correlation between OA and CVD was noted especially among the elderly,[28] another study noted that physically disabled OA patients were more likely to sustain a cardiovascular event compared to non-disabled persons (HR 1.26, 95% CI 1.12–1.42), independent of the presence of clinical and radiographic OA.[29] There is also the question of whether the association of CVD depends on which joint is affected by OA. One study noted that hand OA was associated with a higher risk of developing CVD, whereas those with knee, hip, and spine OA did not.[30,31] In a study that looked at knee OA, there was an association with cardiovascular risk factors such as hypertension and DM, and other Framingham criteria.[32]

Most of the data are derived from epidemiologic studies, and not prospective clinical trials. The differences in findings between population-based studies may be explained by differences in methodology, such as the age of subjects being studied, if patient's functional levels and physiologic musculoskeletal features were included as variables,

Table 6.2 Considerations in assessing medical literature on CVD risk in OA

Subject/patient factors	Age
	Functional levels
	Physiologic musculoskeletal features
	Subject selection (e.g., if OA subjects were selected due to a preexisting diagnosis of CVD, this can lead to potential bias)
CVD factors	Diagnostic methods
	Specific manifestation(s) being studied
OA factors	Diagnostic methods
	Selection of joints affected by OA
Medications	NSAID use – duration of use, discontinuation

Note: CVD, Cardiovascular disease; OA, osteoarthritis; NSAIDs, nonsteroidal anti-inflammatory drugs.

if OA subjects were selected due to a preexisting diagnosis of CVD which then leads to bias, variations in which features of CVD are studied and methods are used to diagnose them, and the differences in how OA is diagnosed and which joints affected by OA are studied (Table 6.2).

Reducing obesity, factoring in disability, and frailty in OA

Reducing obesity is huge endeavor for patients with OA. While increasing physical activity is needed to counter obesity in OA, physical activity is a challenge for patients with severe OA, especially of the hip and knee. OA typically is accompanied by muscle weakness which then imperils physical activity. Muscle weakness is part of the process toward the development of OA, which is of particular significance in regard to quadriceps weakness in knee OA.[33–35]

Further discussion about physical challenges in OA populations warrants an awareness of the concepts of disability and frailty. Disability is the lack of ability to perform an activity in the manner or within the range considered normal for a human being (e.g., capacity to perform tasks as a worker); in contrast functional limitation refers to the inability to perform specific tasks (e.g., inability to walk due to impairments in gait). Frailty is a physiologic concept usually applied in geriatric populations denoted by changes in musculoskeletal, neuroendocrine, and immune systems that lead to functional decline and predisposes to adverse health conditions.[36–38] Disability in older men is related to a function of diminished muscle mass, strength, and performance, and not so much a function of other factors related to body composition, body size and lean mass, and lean mass and weight.[39] Frailty among the elderly has been associated with OA and is marked by a physiologic concept and encompasses decreases in physical activity, muscle strength, overall weakness, fatigue slowness, and weight loss.[37]

Frailty has been linked to CVD, its risk factors, and the incidence of cardiovascular procedures.[40,41] It is elucidated that frailty in elderly populations is associated with elevated acute phase proteins, decreased vitamin D and abnormal levels of sex hormones, cortisol, and growth hormone, myocardial injury, ischemic brain lesions, abnormal ankle–arm ratio, carotid artery stenosis, arterial hypertension, and left ventricular hypertrophy, which are more common in frail patients.[40] It appears that frailty is associated with increased inflammation and elevated levels of blood clotting markers, even when DM and CVD are excluded.[41] Better studies to understand the relationship between disability and frailty in the context of OA and how these directly correlate with increased CVD risk in OA warrant further study.[42]

Inflammation in OA

The causal or pathophysiologic relationship between OA and CVD continues to evolve. The concept of "Inflammageing" has been described as a condition noted by increased inflammation that is linked with chronic morbidity, disability, frailty, and premature death and is a risk factor for CVDs[43]; mechanisms proposed include changes to the microbiome, genetics, inflammasome activation, oxidative stress, immune cell dysregulation, and chronic infections. Inflammageing has also been linked with the development of OA; cartilage degradation and antigens derived from damaged joints may trigger further inflammation through the activation of inflammasomes.[44] In fact, recent advances in OA basic pathophysiology have elucidated an immunopathogenic concept of senescent chondrocytes, and its effects on propagating OA, and pathways leading to its impaired clearance from damaged joints.[45] This has served as the basis for current research in developing immunotherapies for OA, which hopefully will result in clinically feasible and viable options for treatment within the next 10 years.

Management considerations: OA and CVD

NSAIDs, including COX-2 inhibitors, are associated with the development of CVD. With NSAIDs being one of the most common forms of pharmacologic pain management for OA, it is suggested that the increased risk of CVD in OA most likely is related to the use of NSAIDs for OA.[26] With the opioid crisis, reliance on NSAIDs for pain control has increased.[46] However, when risks of CVD are high, it is recommended to avoid NSAIDs. In a study using Swedish registry data of OA patients using NSAIDs, it was found that discontinuation of NSAIDs was associated with reduction in cardiovascular comorbidities.[47] In evaluating the risk of CVD in OA, it is important to consider the use of NSAIDs in this population as a variable.

In conclusion, OA is both a disease involving structural damage of joint tissues and an illness with pain being the predominant symptom. It affects at least 240 million adults worldwide. Evolving concepts on the role of inflammation in OA and its relationship to the development of CVD are emerging and suggest that there is an increased risk for CVD in OA. CVD and OA share common risk factors related to aging and obesity. In general, despite some conflicting data, OA appears to be closely related to the development of CVD. "Inflammageing" is a risk factor for CVD and is associated with increased inflammation leading to chronic morbidity, disability, frailty, and premature death; it also has been linked with the development of OA and it is hypothesized that cartilage degradation and antigens derived from damaged joints may trigger further inflammation through the activation of inflammasomes. Geriatric syndromes related to frailty, and disability, and their association with inflammation and possible links to CVD development deserve further study. Given the inherent risk of CVD with the use of NSAIDs and COX-2 inhibitors, the use of NSAIDs in OA also portends a higher risk of CVD in OA patients, and this variable needs to be considered in evaluating CVD risk in OA.

Acknowledgment

The authors would like to thank Lauren Salinas, Administrator for the Division of Rheumatology at Loma Linda University, for her assistance in preparing the manuscript.

REFERENCES

1. Allen KD, Thoma LM, Golightly YM. Epidemiology of osteoarthritis. *Osteoarthritis Cartilage*. 2022;30(2): 184–195.
2. Yue L, Berman J. What is osteoarthritis? *JAMA*. 2022;327(13):1300.
3. Hunter DJ, Bierma-Zeinstra S. Osteoarthritis. *Lancet*. 2019;393(10182):1745–1759.
4. Katz JN, Arant KR, Loeser RF. Diagnosis and treatment of hip and knee osteoarthritis: a review. *JAMA*. 2021;325(6):568–578.
5. He Y, Li Z, Alexander PG, et al. Pathogenesis of osteoarthritis: risk factors, regulatory pathways in chondrocytes, and experimental models. *Biology*. 2020;9(8):194.
6. Vina ER, Kwoh CK. Epidemiology of osteoarthritis: literature update. *Curr Opin Rheumatol*. 2018;30(2):160–167.
7. Chalian M, Roemer FW, Guermazi A. Advances in osteoarthritis imaging. *Curr Opin Rheumatol*. 2023;35(1):44–54. doi:10.1097/BOR.0000000000000917
8. Kolasinski SL, Neogi T, Hochberg MC, et al. 2019 American College of Rheumatology/ Arthritis Foundation guideline for the management of osteoarthritis of the hand, hip, and knee. *Arthritis Rheumatol*. 2020;72(2):220–233.

9. Kohn MD, Sassoon AA, Fernando ND. Classifications in brief: Kellgren-Lawrence classification of osteoarthritis. *Clin Orthop Relat Res*. 2016;474(8):1886–1893.

10. Swain S, Sarmanova A, Coupland C, Doherty M, Zhang W. Comorbidities in osteoarthritis: a systematic review and meta-analysis of observational studies. *Arthritis Care Res (Hoboken)*. 2020;72(7):991–1000.

11. Sen R, Hurley JA. *Osteoarthritis*. Treasure Island (FL): StatPearls Publishing; February 20, 2023.

12. Watt FE. Posttraumatic osteoarthritis: what have we learned to advance osteoarthritis? *Curr Opin Rheumatol*. 2021;33(1):74–83.

13. Raud B, Gay C, Guiguet-Auclair C, et al. Level of obesity is directly associated with the clinical and functional consequences of knee osteoarthritis. *Sci Rep*. 2020;10(1):3601.

14. Bracilovic A. Why are women more prone to osteoarthritis? *Arthritis Health*. Published January 26, 2021. Accessed February 10, 2023. Available from: https://www.arthritis-health.com/blog/ why-are-women-more-prone-osteoarthritis

15. Punzi L, Galozzi P, Luisetto R, Favero M, Ramonda FO, Scanu A. Post-traumatic arthritis: overview on pathogenic mechanisms and role of inflammation. *RMD Open*. 2016;2(2):e000279.

16. Hawker GA, Lohmander LS. What an earlier recognition of osteoarthritis can do for OA prevention. *Osteoarthritis Cartilage*. 2021;29(12):1632–1634.

17. Obert MR, Vina ER, Bilal J, Kwoh C. "Osteoarthritis." In: Halter JB, Ouslander JG, Studenski S, High KP, Asthana S, Supiano MA, Ritchie CS, Schmader K., eds. *Hazzard's Geriatric Medicine and Gerontology*, 8e. McGraw Hill; 2022.

18. Yusuf E. Pharmacologic and non-pharmacologic treatment of osteoarthritis. *Curr Treat Options Rheumatol*. 2016;2(2):111–125.

19. World Health Organization. Cardiovascular disease. Data and statistics. Accessed April 22, 2023. Available from: https://www.who.int/health-topics/ cardiovascular-diseases#tab=tab_1

20. Gay C, Chabaud A, Guilley E, Coudeyre E. Educating patients about the benefits of physical activity and exercise for their hip and knee osteoarthritis. Systematic literature review. *Ann Phys Rehabil Med*. 2016;59(3):174–183.

21. Raposo F, Ramos M, Lúcia Cruz A. Effects of exercise on knee osteoarthritis: a systematic review. *Musculoskeletal Care*. 2021;19(4):399–435.

22. Gwinnutt JM, Wieczorek M, Rodríguez-Carrio J, et al. Effects of diet on the outcomes of rheumatic and musculoskeletal diseases (RMDs): systematic review and meta-analyses informing the 2021 EULAR recommendations for lifestyle improvements in people with RMDs. *RMD Open*. 2022;8(2):e002167.

23. Ribeiro Rosa K, Fruschein Annichino R, de Azevedo E, Souza Munhoz M, et al. Role of central obesity on pain onset and its association with cardiovascular disease: a retrospective study of a hospital cohort of patients with osteoarthritis. *BMJ Open*. 2022;12(12):e066453.

24. Hall AJ, Stubbs B, Mamas MA, Myint PK, Smith TO. Association between osteoarthritis and cardiovascular disease: systematic review and meta-analysis. *Eur J Prev Cardiol*. 2016;23(9):938–946.

25. Mathieu S, Couderc M, Tournadre A, Soubrier M. Cardiovascular profile in osteoarthritis: a meta-analysis of cardiovascular events and risk factors. *Joint Bone Spine*. 2019;86(6):679–684.

26. Wang H, Bai J, He B, Hu X, Liu D. Osteoarthritis and the risk of cardiovascular disease: a meta-analysis of observational studies. *Sci Rep*. 2016;6:39672.

27. Macêdo MB, Santos VMOS, Pereira RMR, Fuller R. Association between osteoarthritis and atherosclerosis: a systematic review and meta-analysis. *Exp Gerontol*. 2022;161:111734.

28. Rahman MM, Kopec JA, Anis AH, Cibere J, Goldsmith CH. Risk of cardiovascular disease in patients with osteoarthritis: a prospective longitudinal study. *Arthritis Care Res*. 2013;65(12):1951–1958.

29. Hoeven TA, Leening MJ, Bindels PJ, et al. Disability and not osteoarthritis predicts cardiovascular disease: a prospective population-based cohort study. *Ann Rheum Dis*. 2015;74(4):752–756.

30. Veronese N, Trevisan C, De Rui M, et al. Association of osteoarthritis with increased risk of cardiovascular diseases in the elderly: findings from the Progetto Veneto Anziano Study Cohort. *Arthritis Rheumatol.* 2016;68(5):1136–1144.

31. Veronese N, Stubbs B, Solmi M, Smith TO, Reginster JY, Maggi S. Osteoarthristis increases the risk of cardiovascular disease: data from the osteoarthritis initiative. *J Nutr Health Aging.* 2018;22(3):371–376.

32. Kim HS, Shin JS, Lee J, et al. Association between knee osteoarthritis, cardiovascular risk factors, and the Framingham risk score in South Koreans: a cross-sectional study. *PLOS ONE.* 2016;11(10):e0165325.

33. Palmieri-Smith RM, Thomas AC, Karvonen-Gutierrez C, Sowers MF. Isometric quadriceps strength in women with mild, moderate, and severe knee osteoarthritis. *Am J Phys Med Rehabil.* 2010;89(7):541–548.

34. Hootman JM, Macera CA, Ham SA, Helmick CG, Sniezek JE. Physical activity levels among the general US adult population and in adults with and without arthritis. *Arthritis Rheum.* 2003;49(1):129–135.

35. Slemenda C, Heilman DK, Brandt KD, et al. Reduced quadriceps strength relative to body weight: a risk factor for knee osteoarthritis in women? *Arthritis Rheum.* 1998;41(11):1951–1959.

36. National Academies of Sciences, Engineering, and Medicine. Enabling America: Assessing the Role of Rehabilitation Science and Engineering. Washington, DC: The National Academies Press; 1997.

37. Castell MV, van der Pas S, Otero A, et al. Osteoarthritis and frailty in elderly individuals across six European countries: results from the European Project on OSteoArthritis (EPOSA). *BMC Musculoskelet Disord.* 2015;16:359.

38. Pivetta NRS, Marincolo JCS, Neri AL, Aprahamian I, Yassuda MS, Borim FSA. Multimorbidity, frailty and functional disability in octogenarians: a structural equation analysis of relationship. *Arch Gerontol Geriatr.* 2020;86:103931.

39. Zanker J, Blackwell T, Patel S, et al. Factor analysis to determine relative contributions of strength, physical performance, body composition and muscle mass to disability and mobility disability outcomes in older men. *Exp Gerontol.* 2022;161:111714.

40. Wleklik M, Denfeld Q, Lisiak M, et al. Frailty syndrome in older adults with cardiovascular diseases-what do we know and what requires further research? *Int J Environ Res Public Health.* 2022;19(4):2234.

41. Walston J, McBurnie MA, Newman A, et al. Frailty and activation of the inflammation and coagulation systems with and without clinical comorbidities: results from the Cardiovascular Health Study. *Arch Intern Med.* 2002;162(20):2333–2341.

42. Espinoza SE, Quiben M, Hazuda HP. Distinguishing comorbidity, disability, and frailty. *Curr Geriatr Rep.* 2018;7(4):201–209.

43. Ferrucci L, Fabbri E. Inflammageing: chronic inflammation in ageing, cardiovascular disease, and frailty. *Nat Rev Cardiol.* 2018;15(9):505–522.

44. Motta F, Barone E, Sica A, Selmi C. Inflammaging and osteoarthritis. *Clin Rev Allergy Immunol.* 2023;64(2):222–238. doi:10.1007/s12016-022-08941-1

45. Liu Y, Zhang Z, Li T, Xu H, Zhang H. Senescence in osteoarthritis: from mechanism to potential treatment. *Arthritis Res Ther.* 2022;24(1):174.

46. Thorlund JB, Turkiewicz A, Prieto-Alhambra D, Englund M. Opioid use in knee or hip osteoarthritis: a region-wide population-based cohort study. *Osteoarthritis Cartilage.* 2019;27(6):871–877.

47. Dell'Isola A, Turkiewicz A, Zhang W, et al. Does osteoarthritis modify the association between NSAID use and risk of comorbities and adverse events? *Osteoarthr Cartil Open.* 2022;4(2):100253.

7

Cardiovascular disease in systemic lupus erythematosus and antiphospholipid antibody syndrome

KARINA D. TORRALBA, NOELLE A. ROLLE, AND VANEET K. SANDHU

INTRODUCTION

Cardiovascular diseases (CVD) are predominant causes of morbidity and mortality in rheumatic diseases, especially in systemic lupus erythematosus (SLE) and antiphospholipid syndrome (APS). Both are autoimmune diseases predominantly affecting premenopausal women. SLE is characterized by multisystem organ manifestations and the presence of autoantibodies and immune complex formation, whereas APS is characterized by thrombotic vascular events and the presence of antiphospholipid antibodies (aPL). Approximately half of SLE patients may develop APS during their disease course while a third of APS patients have SLE.[1,2]

The concern for CVD is significant in many rheumatic diseases, with a particular emphasis on its significance in SLE and APS. The European Alliance of Associations for Rheumatology (EULAR) has recently responded to this concern by issuing guidelines addressing these issues (summarized in Table 7.1).[3] In SLE, the risk of stroke and myocardial infarction (MI) is reported to be two to three times higher than that in the general population.[4] Premenopausal women aged 35–44 with SLE face a staggering 52-fold increase in the risk of MI,

notably occurring at least ten years earlier than the general population at risk for MI.[5] Valvular heart disease (VHD) affects up to 15% of patients with APS and is associated with an increased risk of stroke.[6]

Traditional and SLE-specific risk factors are listed in Table 7.2. Traditional risk factors such as hypertension and diabetes alone do not entirely explain the heightened risk of CVD in SLE. The fact that CVD, typically an uncommon cause of mortality in young females, becomes a predominant cause in SLE, especially in the later stages of the disease, implies that there are other factors related to SLE itself and its treatment that contributes to the risk of developing CVD. Longer disease duration and highly active disease are linked to the development of CVD.[7,8] Carotid plaques, indicative of future cardiovascular events, are associated with higher disease activity and damage scores as well as lupus nephritis.[7] Lupus nephritis is further associated with a higher prevalence of plaques, MI, and stroke.[9,10] Steroids, used to treat SLE flares, exhibit an association with increased rates of cardiovascular events, particularly when given for prolonged periods at doses of 7.5 mg or more daily prednisone equivalent.[11]

DOI: 10.1201/9781003386711-7

Table 7.1 Cardiovascular disease management and risk factors in SLE and APS

SLE

- Assess traditional CVR and SLE-related factors
- BP Target <130/80
- Nephritis – ACE inhibitors, ARBs in UPCr >500mg/g or arterial hypertension
- Preventive strategies (e.g. LDA)
- No prior thrombosis but high- or low-risk aPL profile: Consider pLDA
- Low SLE disease activity = low CVR
- Lowest possible corticosteroid dose
- No specific immunosuppression to lower the risk of CVE
- Hydroxychloroquine should be considered to reduce CVE

APS

- Assess traditional CVR & SLE-related factors
- BP management – follow general population recommendations
- Asymptomatic aPL carriers with high-risk aPL profile with/without traditional risk factors: Consider pLDA

CVR: cardiovascular risk, ACE: angiotensin-converting enzymes, ARBs: angiotensin receptor blockers, UPCr: urine protein/creatinine ratio, LDA: low-dose aspirin, pLDA: prophylactic low-dose aspirin, CVE: cardiovascular events, aPL: antiphospholipid antibody

Source: Adapted from 2022 EULAR guidelines.[3]

Table 7.2 Cardiovascular disease risk factors

Major independent risk factors

Cigarette smoking	Low serum HDL
Elevated blood pressure	cholesterol
Elevated serum total	Diabetes mellitus
and LDL cholesterol	Advancing age

Other (predisposing) risk factors

Obesity	Family history of
Abdominal obesity	premature CHD
Physical inactivity	Ethnic characteristics
	Psychosocial factors

Conditional risk factors

Elevated serum	Elevated serum
triglycerides	lipoprotein(a)
Small LDL particles	Prothrombotic factors
Elevated serum	(e.g. fibrinogen)
homocysteine	Inflammatory markers
	(e.g. C-reactive)

Lupus-specific risk factors

Dysregulation of	Greater damage
innate/adaptive	accrual
immune systems	Chronic use of
Older age at diagnosis	corticosteroids
High disease activity	Use of non-steroidal
Longer duration of	anti-inflammatory
disease	drugs
	Lupus nephritis

APS-specific risk factors

Antiphospholipid	Platelet activation
antibodies	Medications
Endothelial dysfunction	

Source: Adapted from Grundy et al.[76]

PATHOGENIC MECHANISMS OF CVD IN SLE AND APS

Endothelial dysfunction, characterized by a diminished ability for vasodilation in the presence of inflammation and thrombosis, has been identified in SLE patients, suggesting a predisposition to CVD.[12] Impaired endothelial cell death and increased apoptosis, along with elevated levels of type 1 interferon, have also been observed.[13,14] Arterial stiffness, contributing to heightened pulse pressures and CVD, has found to be elevated in SLE compared to controls.[12]

Alterations in lipid profiles, marked by high total cholesterol, very low-density lipoprotein (VLDL), triglycerides (TG), and decreased or dysfunctional high-density lipoprotein (HDL), have been observed in active SLE.[15–17] Reduced lipoprotein lipase (LPL) activity due to autoantibodies, resulting in increased TG, has been associated with heightened SLE activity.[16] Disruptions in apolipoprotein C-III, angiopoietin-like protein 4, and LPL have been observed in SLE patients, with increased damage correlating with higher serum levels of LPL.[18]

Foam cell formation in SLE occurs due to impaired cholesterol efflux capacity caused by the loss of HDL activity to inhibit LDL oxidation.[19] Low-density granulocytes, an inflammatory set of neutrophils that have a higher tendency to form neutrophil extracellular traps (NETs), can cause lipoprotein oxidation.[20] A comprehensive review of these pathogenic mechanisms in SLE[21] and APS[22] has been described in detail.

MAJOR CARDIAC MANIFESTATIONS OF SLE

The leading cause of death in SLE is cardiac involvement, affecting more than 50% of patients and impacting any region of the heart.[23]

Pericardial disease

Pericardial involvement is the most common echocardiographic lesion in SLE and is the most frequent cause of symptomatic cardiac disease (11–57%).[24–26] Pericardial effusion occurs in more than 50% of patients with SLE at some point in their disease course, and pericarditis may precede many other clinical signs of the disease.

Pericardial disease may be asymptomatic and discovered incidentally during imaging performed for other reasons. When symptomatic, patients may present with pleuritic chest pain, dyspnea, palpitations, and fatigue. On examination, findings may include a friction rub on auscultation.[23] Signs of serositis elsewhere, such as pleural effusions and ascites, may also be present. Pericardial effusions are typically small, and cardiac tamponade is rare. However, 5–13% of hospitalized patients with symptomatic pericarditis may progress to develop tamponade. Recurrence of pericarditis after the first episode is noted in 15–30% of cases, with constrictive and purulent pericarditis representing other rarely reported complications.[25,27]

The presence of anti-Smith antibodies and anti-dsDNA antibodies is associated with lupus pericarditis. Electrocardiogram (ECG) may reveal diffuse ST elevations or PR depressions and echocardiogram may reveal a pericardial effusion or a thickened pericardium. Complement and immune complex deposition are noted in a granular pattern on direct immunofluorescence.[28]

Myocardial disease

Myocarditis is often an asymptomatic manifestation of SLE and is present in 8–25% of SLE patients. Through the use of cardiac MRI, asymptomatic myocardial abnormalities were observed in 43%

of SLE patients. Risk is higher in Black populations compared to Caucasian and Hispanic populations.[29,30] Myocarditis should be suspected in patients exhibiting symptoms of congestive heart failure (CHF), such as dyspnea, tachycardia not easily explained by another underlying cause, chest pain, fever, and palpitations.

Laboratory abnormalities include elevated ESR, low C3/C4, and elevated troponin levels. There may be ECG abnormalities or unexplained cardiomegaly. Echocardiography may reveal abnormalities in both systolic and diastolic function of the left ventricle and global or patchy hypokinesis not in a specific coronary artery distribution. In instances where inflammation has led to fibrosis, the patient may clinically manifest as dilated cardiomyopathy.

Cardiac MRI using T2-related images demonstrates delayed gadolinium enhancement, although this is not specific to SLE-associated myocarditis. To confirm, right heart catheterization (RHC) with endometrial biopsy will show infiltration of the myocardium with mononuclear cells. Autopsy findings indicate that 57% of SLE patients have myocarditis.[31]

The majority of lupus myocarditis patients require care in an intensive care unit setting. Despite treatment, mortality rates range from 4 to 10%. If left untreated, myocarditis may lead to arrhythmias, conduction abnormalities, CHF, and an increased risk of sudden cardiac death.

Myocarditis may accompany pericarditis and may also be attributed to drugs or other comorbidities. Additional etiologies to consider in the differential diagnosis of lupus myocarditis include MI, vasculitis, and CHF.

Valvular disease

Unlike many other manifestations of SLE that are more frequent and severe during flares of disease activity, valvular lesions in SLE may occur at any time, and their presence usually does not correlate with disease activity. Valvular involvement in SLE includes mitral valve prolapse (MVP) and Libman–Sacks endocarditis also called nonbacterial thrombotic endocarditis (NBTE) or verrucous endocarditis.[32]

Patients are typically asymptomatic, but in rare cases, VHD in SLE may present with dyspnea and features of left-sided CHF. MVP appears to occur more frequently in patients with SLE, with estimates suggesting its occurrence in 21% of SLE cases compared to 5.5% of controls.[33] Libman and Sacks described four cases of NBTE in 1924, and today its prevalence can be found in 11–74% of SLE patients.[32] The most commonly affected valve is the mitral valve followed by the atrial valve.

VHD is more prevalent in patients with significantly elevated levels of aPL.[34] A high index of suspicion for VHD should be kept in mind for SLE patients with these antibodies, and routine cardiac auscultation should be performed. Echocardiogram consideration is warranted for patients with murmurs or changing cardiac function. While it is believed that aPL can cause platelet aggregation leading to thrombus formation, a secondary theory suggests that immune complex deposition on valvular tissues leads to inflammatory infiltration.

Patients with SLE are at an increased risk for infection due to their immunocompromised state. It is therefore imperative to consider bacterial endocarditis in a patient presenting with fever and a new murmur. The diagnostic evaluation should include blood cultures and echocardiography.

Conduction abnormalities

The most common conduction abnormalities in patients with SLE are sinus tachycardia (18%), QT prolongation (17%), and atrial fibrillation (9%).[35] These abnormalities may be secondary to active myocarditis or a history thereof. While there has been a suggestion of an association between anti-Ro/SSA antibodies and QT prolongation in adults, this has not been confirmed in larger studies.[32]

Congestive heart failure

SLE is a significant cause of CHF in the young, stemming from cardiac inflammation involving the myocardium, valves, and conduction abnormalities. As the disease progresses, atherosclerosis and coronary artery disease (CAD) contribute to 29% of CHF cases in SLE. Renal involvement in SLE is correlated with earlier and higher incidence of CHF. The absolute ten-year risk of CHF in SLE patients was 3.71% compared to 1.94% in controls. SLE patients who subsequently develop CHF experience higher mortality rates compared to CHF in populations without SLE.[36]

Pulmonary arterial hypertension

Pulmonary arterial hypertension (PAH), previously thought to be rare, apparently has a prevalence to be 2.6–3.8% in SLE populations.[37] Patients can present with progressive exertional dyspnea and fatigue, and diagnosis is often delayed. Several disease-related factors have been associated with the presence of PAH such as Raynaud's phenomenon, history of serositis, APS antibodies, and anti-RNP antibodies.[38]

Neonatal lupus and congenital heart block

Infants with neonatal lupus sometimes develop complete heart block (CHB), a condition that may necessitate pacing for survival.[32] CHB may be present in fetuses or neonates born to mothers with elevated titers of anti-Ro or anti-La antibodies, even among those who do not have SLE. It is believed that damage to the fetal heart is induced by the binding of maternal anti-Ro/anti-La antibodies to apoptotic cardiocytes, thereby impairing appropriate removal by healthy cardiocytes in embryogenesis.[39] While this antibody is estimated to be present in approximately 40% of SLE patients,[40] the risk of having a child with CHB is about 2%.[41] If an anti-Ro/SSA antibody-positive mother previously had a child with CHB, the risk increases to >15%.[42]

The onset of complications in neonatal lupus occurs in the mid-to-late second trimester, coinciding with two critical processes: Placental transfer of maternal antibodies and development of the fetal cardiac conduction system. Pregnant SLE patients with anti-Ro/anti-La antibodies should be followed closely with fetal echocardiography at 16 or 18 weeks through 28 weeks at 1–2 week intervals.[42]

CARDIAC MANIFESTATIONS OF APS

A combination of various pathophysiologic processes, including endothelial dysfunction with proliferation and intimal hyperplasia, atherogenesis, platelet activation, inflammation, and dysregulation of coagulation-fibrinolysis, appears to predispose patients with APS to cardiac disease.[43]

Valvular heart disease

VHD occurs in approximately one-third of patients with APS, with a tendency to damage the mitral valve.[44] It can manifest as NBTE and valvular dysfunction. Immune complexes causing damage to the valvular endothelium with resulting fibrotic changes are thought to be the underlying process of VHD in APS.[6] Severe heart valve disease increases the risk of stroke. Heart valve replacement surgery is needed in 5% of patients and can be complicated by bleeding and thrombosis.[45]

Myocardial infarction

Acute MI may be the presenting feature of APS, typically in younger individuals and at increased frequency when secondary to SLE.[46] Ischemia is believed to be a result of accelerated atherosclerosis, microvascular dysfunction, and/or thromboembolic disease.[47] Multiple studies have demonstrated independent risk factors for MI in those with elevated titers of aPL with or without APS.[48] Traditional cardiovascular disease diagnostic tools, including coronary angiography, may appear unremarkable.

Myocardial dysfunction

While less frequently reported, myocardial dysfunction may occur in APS as a result of antibodies in the myocardium causing ventricular dysfunction or coronary artery or microvascular thrombosis.[49] Echocardiogram may reveal myocardial dysfunction in both primary and secondary APS with a more severe right ventricular diastolic impairment in primary APS compared to secondary disease.[50] Late gadolinium enhancement and lower myocardial perfusion reserve are noted on positron emission tomography. Positron emission tomography studies in APS populations reveal a higher prevalence of late gadolinium enhancement and lower myocardial perfusion reserve.[51,52]

Other less common cardiac manifestations of APS include PAH and intracardiac thrombosis. While venous thromboembolism is common in APS, and pulmonary embolism due to APS may lead to chronic thromboembolic pulmonary hypertension, the prevalence and risk factors for pulmonary hypertension in APS warrant further evaluation.

OTHER CLINICAL CONSIDERATIONS

Cardiac disease in SLE transplant patients

It is not unusual for SLE patients to undergo organ transplantation when irreversible damage is incurred due to severe disease activity.

Approximately 20% of SLE patients progress to end-stage renal disease requiring organ transplantation. Survival rates for SLE patients up to 10 years post-renal transplant are up to 75%.[53] Renal transplantation is associated with reduced risk of cardiovascular events, including MI and stroke.[54] However, SLE patients who receive kidney transplants have a lower survival rate than control patients, and the mortality is due to cardiovascular events.[55]

Cardiac transplants among SLE patients are much less common, possibly due to the concerns by some transplant centers regarding the recurrence of heart disease. Currently, there are no registry or other studies to address the issue of heart disease post-heart transplant in SLE patients. However, case reports have noted good outcomes.[56]

In general, there are concerns regarding the cardiovascular toxicity of immunosuppressive medications used post-transplant, particularly in regard to their mechanistic effects noted in pre-clinical studies. However, due to a discordance with clinical data, further translational studies are needed to clarify this issue.[57]

Pregnancy and heart disease in lupus

A meta-analysis of studies spanning from 2001 to 2016 confirms that SLE patients do experience a high impact on maternal and fetal outcomes following pregnancy.[58] Maternal outcomes included pre-eclampsia, hypertension, and postpartum infection, while fetal outcomes included premature birth and restrictions on fetal growth. The use of hydroxychloroquine (HCQ) during pregnancy has been shown to mitigate these effects.[59]

A literature search specifically focusing on CVD occurring during pregnancy in SLE patients reveals limited information. Similarly, there is a lack of literature addressing pregnancy outcomes among SLE patients with preexisting cardiac manifestations.

In-stent restenosis risk in SLE

In-stent restenosis (ISR) is an anomalous process of repair whereby there are an increased number of vascular smooth muscle cells, along with excessive extracellular proteoglycans and type III collagen. SLE patients, like other patients with autoimmune diseases, appear to have higher rates of ISR compared to the general population, which is attributed to the underlying endothelial dysfunction present in inflammatory autoimmune diseases.[60] Animal models have shown that the use of methotrexate and anti-tumor necrosis factor agents can reduce ISR.

COVID-19-related concerns: CVD in SLE

A global registry has noted that the presence of CVD is one of the many factors that drive severe outcomes among patients with SLE who have COVID-19 infection.[61] In looking at rheumatic diseases in general, corticosteroid use at a dose of ≥10 mg/day prednisone equivalent was associated with higher rates of hospitalization, while the use of steroid-sparing immunomodulators was not; there was no reduced risk observed with the use of HCQ.[62] CVD was one of the independent risk factors associated with COVID-19-related death.[63]

COVID-19 vaccination has been associated with the development of CVDs,[64,65] with myocarditis being reported to be the most common manifestation with the use of mRNA vaccines.[66]

A comprehensive review of 198 studies demonstrated that SLE patients have a higher risk of acquiring COVID-19 infection, with elevated rates of hospitalization, severity, and death than the general population. COVID-19 vaccines are considered relatively safe for SLE patients, with minimal risk of severe flares. Additionally, the attitudes of SLE patients toward vaccination were predominantly positive.[67]

Cardiac effects of treatments

HCQ has been one of the mainstay treatments for SLE for decades. Although generally well tolerated, it gained significant attention during the COVID-19 pandemic. A study evaluating the relationship between HCQ drug levels and adverse effects, as well as disease activity scores in rheumatic diseases, including SLE, revealed that HCQ levels correlate with QTc prolongation.[68]

Cyclophosphamide, through its metabolite acrolein, has been associated with left ventricular dysfunction and heart failure in the oncology literature. However, cyclophosphamide is usually given in combination with other medications such as anthracyclines (doxorubicin) which have well-established cardiotoxic effects.[69] A search of the literature looking at cardiotoxicity associated with cyclophosphamide treatment for SLE did not reveal relevant results.

CVD MANAGEMENT IN SLE AND APS

The EULAR guidelines on the management of cardiovascular risk factors in rheumatic diseases including SLE and APLS[3] emphasize the use of cardiovascular risk prediction tools, interventions on traditional factors, and the importance of controlling disease activity and minimizing damage. While many recommendations were based on expert opinion due to a lack of high-level evidence, these guidelines serve as a nidus for further research in this field. SLE-specific recommendations included a blood pressure target of <130/80 mm Hg, antiplatelet use, disease activity control, corticosteroid minimization, and HCQ use to reduce risk.

The use of aspirin in SLE and APS patients at high risk of thrombosis (Table 7.1) is endorsed due to protective antiplatelet effects that prevent atherothrombosis. However, the EULAR guidelines emphasize that the use of aspirin for primary prevention of cardiovascular in other disease states (i.e. scleroderma, Sjögren's syndrome) may not be necessary unless other medical conditions exist that warrant its use.[3]

There is substantial literature supporting the protective role of HCQ against CVD in SLE including six cohort studies demonstrating that HCQ use lowers the risk of atherothrombotic events.[3,70] HCQ has also been shown to prevent recurrent thrombosis and miscarriages in APS.[71]

Colchicine is a potent anti-inflammatory drug which inhibits inhibiting microtubule polymerization, reduces the production of pro-inflammatory cytokines including IL-1B, and inhibits neutrophil chemotaxis. Adverse events associated with colchicine use include gastrointestinal intolerance and myopathy. Caution should be exercised when taking colchicine with other drugs that inhibits or induces the cytochrome p450 enzyme system. Historically, it has been used for pericarditis patients in general, but there is evidence suggesting its utility in SLE-related pericarditis.[72] Larger, long-term studies are needed to further evaluate its efficacy and risk profile.

Further understanding the pathophysiologic pathways leading to pericarditis and SLE in general has led to the development of treatments directed toward specific immunologic targets.

Biologic IL-1 inhibitors have been used for refractory pericarditis, particularly for autoinflammatory syndromes. Rilonacept, the first inhibitor of both IL1-α and β, has been approved for use in pericarditis. Studies are needed to demonstrate the efficacy and safety of IL-1 inhibitors for lupus pericarditis.[73]

Belimumab is a fully humanized IgG1γ monoclonal antibody directed against soluble B lymphocyte stimulator (BLyS). Long-term data show that it reduces accumulation of organ damage, number of flares, and corticosteroid use.[74] Further studies are needed to investigate the specific beneficial effects of Belimumab on CVD in SLE.

Anifrolumab is a monoclonal antibody targeting the type I interferon α receptor FDA-approved for the treatment of SLE. Long-term data indicate that its use was associated with lower cumulative glucocorticoid use, greater mean improvement in the SLE Disease Activity Index 2000, and no significant major cardiovascular events, when compared with placebo.[75] Its direct effects on lupus-related cardiac disease need further study. It remains to be seen if its steroid-sparing effect also translates to decreased cardiovascular events in SLE populations as compared with patients who remain on corticosteroids.

REFERENCES

1. Petri M. Epidemiology of the antiphospholipid antibody syndrome. *J Autoimmun.* 2000 Sep;15(2):145–151.
2. Cervera R. Lessons from the "Euro-Phospholipid" project. *Autoimmun Rev.* 2008 Jan;7(3):174–178.
3. Drosos GC, Vedder D, Houben E, et al. EULAR recommendations for cardiovascular risk management in rheumatic and musculoskeletal diseases, including systemic lupus erythematosus and antiphospholipid syndrome. *Ann Rheum Dis.* 2022;81(6):768–779.
4. Yazdany J, Pooley N, Langham J, et al. Systemic lupus erythematosus; stroke and myocardial infarction risk: a systematic review and meta-analysis. *RMD Open.* 2020 Sep;6(2):e001247.
5. Manzi S, Meilahn EN, Rairie JE, et al. Age-specific incidence rates of myocardial infarction and angina in women with systemic lupus erythematosus: comparison with the Framingham study. *Am J Epidemiol.* 1997;145:408–415.
6. Kolitz T, Shiber S, Sharabi I, et al. Cardiac manifestations of antiphospholipid syndrome with focus on its primary form. *Front Immunol.* 2019;10:941.
7. Roman MJ, Shanker BA, Davis A, et al. Prevalence and correlates of accelerated atherosclerosis in systemic lupus erythematosus. *N Engl J Med.* 2003;349:2399–2406.
8. Chen J, Tang Y, Zhu M, Xu A. Heart involvement in systemic lupus erythematosus: a systemic review and meta-analysis. *Clin Rheumatol.* 2016;35:2437–2448.
9. Stojan G, Li J, Budoff M, et al. High-risk coronary plaque in SLE: low-attenuation non-calcified coronary plaque and positive remodeling index. *Lupus Sci Med.* 2020 Jul;7(1):e000409.
10. Gustafsson JT, Herlitz Lindberg M, et al. Excess atherosclerosis in systemic lupus erythematosus – a matter of renal involvement: case control study of 281 SLE patients and 281 individually matched population controls. *PLOS ONE.* 2017;12:e0174572.
11. Al Sawah S, Zhang X, Zhu B, et al. Effect of corticosteroid use by dose on the risk of developing organ damage over time in systemic Lupus erythematosus-the Hopkins Lupus Cohort. *Lupus Sci Med.* 2015;2(1):e000066.
12. Mendoza-Pinto C, Rojas-Villarraga A, Molano-Gonzalez N, et al. Endothelial dysfunction, and arterial stiffness in patients with systemic lupus erythematosus: a systematic review and meta-analysis. *Atherosclerosis.* 2020;297:55–63.

13. Rajagopalan S, Somers EC, Brook RD, et al. Endothelial cell apoptosis in systemic lupus erythematosus: a common pathway for abnormal vascular function and thrombosis propensity. *Blood*. 2004;103:3677–3683.

14. Lee PY, Li Y, Richards HB, Chan FS, et al. Type I interferon as a novel risk factor for endothelial progenitor cell depletion and endothelial dysfunction in systemic lupus erythematosus. *Arthritis Rheum*. 2007;56:3759–3769.

15. Tselios K, Koumaras C, Gladman DD, Urowitz MB. Dyslipidemia in systemic lupus erythematosus: just another comorbidity? *Semin Arthritis Rheum*. 2016;45:604–610.

16. de Carvalho JF, Borba EF, Viana VS, et al. Anti-lipoprotein lipase antibodies: a new player in the complex atherosclerotic process in systemic lupus erythematosus? *Arthritis Rheum*. 2004;50:3610–3615.

17. McMahon M, Grossman J, Skaggs B, et al. Dysfunctional proinflammatory high-density lipoproteins confer increased risk of atherosclerosis in women with systemic lupus erythematosus. *Arthritis Rheum*. 2009;60:2428–2437.

18. Quevedo-Abeledo JC, Martín-González C, Ferrer-Moure C, et al. Key molecules of triglycerides pathway metabolism are disturbed in patients with systemic lupus erythematosus. *Front Immunol*. 2022;9(13):827355.

19. Ronda N, Favari E, Borghi MO, et al. Impaired serum cholesterol efflux capacity in rheumatoid arthritis and systemic lupus erythematosus. *Ann Rheum Dis*. 2014;73:609–615.

20. Carlucci PM, Purmalek MM, Dey AK, et al. Neutrophil subsets and their gene signature associate with vascular inflammation and coronary atherosclerosis in lupus. *JCI Insight*. 2018;3(8):e99276.

21. Oliveira CB, Kaplan MJ. Cardiovascular disease risk and pathogenesis in systemic lupus erythematosus. *Semin Immunopathol*. 2022;44(3):309–324.

22. Tektonidou MG. Cardiovascular disease risk in antiphospholipid syndrome: thrombo-inflammation and atherothrombosis. *J Autoimmun*. 2022;128:102813.

23. Zagelbaum Ward NK, Linars-Koloffon D, Posligua A, et al. Cardiac manifestations of systemic lupus erythematous: an overview of the incidence, risk factors, diagnostic criteria, pathophysiology and treatment options. *Cardiol Rev*. 2022;30(1):38–43.

24. Man BL, Mok CC. Serositis related to systemic lupus erythematosus: prevalence and outcome. *Lupus*. 2005;14(10): 822–826.

25. Rosenbaum E, Krebs E, Cohen M, Tiliakos A, Derk CT. The spectrum of clinical manifestations, outcome, and treatment of pericardial tamponade in patients with systemic lupus erythematosus: a retrospective study and literature review. *Lupus*. 2009;18(7):608–612.

26. Ryu S, Fu W, Petri MA. Associates and predictors of pleurisy or pericarditis in SLE. *Lupus Sci Med*. 2017 Oct 23;4(1):e000221.

27. Goswami RP, Sircar G, Ghosh A, Ghosh P. Cardiac tamponade in systemic lupus erythematosus. *QJM*. 2018;111:83.

28. Tincani A, Rebaioli CB, Taglietti M, et al. Heart involvement in systemic lupus erythematosus, anti-phospholipid syndrome and neonatal lupus. *Rheumatology (Oxford)*. 2006;45:iv8–13.

29. Apte M, McGwin G Jr, Vilá LM, et al. Associated factors and impact of myocarditis in patients with SLE from LUMINA, a multiethnic US cohort (LV) [corrected]. *Rheumatology (Oxford)*. 2008;47:362.

30. du Toit R, Karamchand S, Doubell AF, et al. Lupus myocarditis: review of current diagnostic modalities and their application in clinical practice. *Rheumatology (Oxford)*. 2023;62:523.

31. Wijetunga M, Rockson S. Myocarditis in systemic lupus erythematosus. *Am J Med*. 2002 Oct 1;113(5):419–423.

32. Miner JJ, Kim AH. Cardiac manifestations of systemic lupus erythematosus. *Rheum Dis Clin North Am*. 2014;40:51.

33. Evangelopoulos ME, Alevizaki M, Toumanidis S, et al. Mitral valve prolapse in systemic lupus erythematosus patients: clinical and immunological aspects. *Lupus*. 2003;12:308.

34. Zuily S, Regnault V, Selton-Suty C, et al. Increased risk for heart valve disease associated with antiphospholipid antibodies in

patients with systemic lupus erythematosus: meta-analysis of echocardiographic studies. *Circulation*. 2011;124:215.

35. Myung G, Forbess LJ, Ishimori ML, et al. Prevalence of resting-ECG abnormalities in systemic lupus erythematosus: a single-center experience. *Clin Rheumatol*. 2017;36:1311.

36. Yafasova A, Fosbøl EL, Schou M, et al. Long-term cardiovascular outcomes in systemic lupus erythematosus. *J Am Coll Cardiol*. 2021;77(14):1717–1727.

37. Pérez-Peñate GM, Rúa-Figueroa I, Juliá-Serdá G, et al. Pulmonary arterial hypertension in systemic lupus erythematosus: prevalence and predictors. *J Rheumatol*. 2016;43(2):323–329.

38. Tani C, Elefante E, Arnaud L, et al. Rare clinical manifestations in systemic lupus erythematosus: a review on frequency and clinical presentation. *Clin Exp Rheumatol*. 2022;40 Suppl 134(5):93–102.

39. Clancy RM, Neufing PJ, Zheng P, et al. Impaired clearance of apoptotic cardiocytes is linked to anti-SSA/Ro and -SSB/La antibodies in the pathogenesis of congenital heart block. *J Clin Invest*. 2006;116(9):2413–2422.

40. Keogan M, Kearns G, Jefferies CA. "Extractable nuclear antigens and SLE: Specificity and role in disease pathogenesis." In: Systemic Lupus Erythematosus, 5th ed. Lahita RG, Tsokos G, Buyon J, Koike T (Eds), 2011 (p. 259). Academic Press, San Diego.

41. Brucato A, Frassi M, Franceschini F, et al. Risk of congenital complete heart block in newborns of mothers with anti-Ro/SSA antibodies detected by counterimmunoelectrophoresis: a prospective study of 100 women. *Arthritis Rheum*. 2001;44(8):1832.

42. Donofrio MT, Moon-Grady AJ, Hornberger LK et al. American Heart Association Adults with Congenital Heart Disease Joint Committee of the Council on Cardiovascular Disease in the Young and Council on Clinical Cardiology, Council on Cardiovascular Surgery and Anesthesia, and Council on Cardiovascular and Stroke Nursing. Diagnosis and treatment of fetal cardiac disease: a scientific statement from the American Heart Association. *Circulation*. 2014;129(21):2183–2242.

43. Polytarchou K, Varvarousis D, Manolis AS. Cardiovascular disease in antiphospholipid syndrome. *Curr Vasc Pharmacol*. 2020;18(6):538–548.

44. Nesher G, Ilany J, Rosenmann D, Abraham AS. Valvular dysfunction in antiphospholipid syndrome: prevalence, clinical features, and treatment. *Semin Arthritis Rheum*. 1997;27(1):27–35.

45. Zuily S, Huttin O, Mohamed S, et al. Valvular heart disease in antiphospholipid syndrome. *Curr Rheumatol Rep*. 2013;15(4):320.

46. Cervera R, Piette JC, Font J, Khamashta MA, Shoenfeld Y, Camps MT, et al. Antiphospholipid syndrome: clinical and immunologic manifestations and patterns of disease expression in a cohort of 1,000 patients. *Arthritis Rheum*. 2002;46:1019–1027.

47. Nazir S, Tachamo N, Lohani S, et al. Acute myocardial infarction and antiphospholipid antibody syndrome: a systematic review. *Coron Artery Dis*. 2017;28:332–335.

48. Shoenfeld Y, Gerli R, Doria A, Matsuura E, Cerinic MM, Ronda N, et al. Accelerated atherosclerosis in autoimmune rheumatic diseases. *Circulation*. 2005;112:3337–3347.

49. Lauwerys BR, Lambert M, Vanoverschelde JL, et al. Myocardial microangiopathy associated with antiphospholipid antibodies. *Lupus*. 2001;10:123–125.

50. Kampolis C, Tektonidou M, Moyssakis I, et al. Evolution of cardiac dysfunction in patients with antiphospholipid antibodies and/or antiphospholipid syndrome: a 10-year follow-up study. *Semin Arthritis Rheum*. 2014;43:558–565.

51. Sacré K, Brihaye B, Hyafil F, et al. Asymptomatic myocardial ischemic disease in antiphospholipid syndrome: a controlled cardiac magnetic resonance imaging study. *Arthritis Rheum*. 2010;62(7):2093–2100.

52. Mavrogeni SI, Markousis-Mavrogenis G, Karapanagiotou O, et al. Silent myocardial perfusion abnormalities detected by stress cardiovascular magnetic resonance in antiphospholipid syndrome: a case-control study. *J Clin Med*. 2019;8(7):1084.

53. Considine SW, Davis NF, McLoughlin LC, et al. Long-term outcomes of renal transplant in patients with end-stage renal failure due to systemic lupus erythematosus and granulomatosis with polyangiitis. *Exp Clin Transplant*. 2019;17(6):720–726.

54. Jorge A, Fu X, Cook C, et al. Kidney transplantation and cardiovascular events among patients with end-stage renal disease due to lupus nephritis: a nationwide cohort study. *Arthritis Care Res (Hoboken)*. 2022;74(11):1829–1834.

55. Norby GE, Leivestad T, Mjøen G, et al. Premature cardiovascular disease in patients with systemic lupus erythematosus influences survival after renal transplantation. *Arthritis Rheum*. 2011 Mar;63(3):733–737.

56. Chapa JJ, Ilonze OJ, Guglin ME, et al. Heart transplantation in systemic lupus erythematosus: a case report and meta-analysis. *Heart Lung*. 2022;52:174–181.

57. Elezaby A, Dexheimer R, Sallam K. Cardiovascular effects of immunosuppression agents. *Front Cardiovasc Med*. 2022 Sep 21;9:981838.

58. Bundhun PK, Soogund MZ, Huang F. Impact of systemic lupus erythematosus on maternal and fetal outcomes following pregnancy: a meta-analysis of studies published between years 2001–2016. *J Autoimmun*. 2017 May;79:17–27.

59. Duan J, Ma D, Wen X, et al. Hydroxychloroquine prophylaxis for preeclampsia, hypertension and prematurity in pregnant patients with systemic lupus erythematosus: a meta-analysis. *Lupus*. 2021;30(7):1163–1174.

60. Pepe M, Napoli G, Carulli E, et al. Autoimmune diseases in patients undergoing percutaneous coronary intervention: a risk factor for in-stent restenosis? *Atherosclerosis*. 2021;333:24–31.

61. Ugarte-Gil MF, Alarcón GS, Izadi Z, et al. Characteristics associated with poor COVID-19 outcomes in individuals with systemic lupus erythematosus: data from the COVID-19 Global Rheumatology Alliance. *Ann Rheum Dis*. 2022;81(7):970–978.

62. Gianfrancesco M, Hyrich KL, Al-Adely S, et al. Characteristics associated with hospitalisation for COVID-19 in people with rheumatic disease: data from the COVID-19 Global Rheumatology Alliance physician-reported registry. *Ann Rheum Dis*. 2020 Jul;79(7):859–866.

63. Strangfeld A, Schäfer M, Gianfrancesco MA, et al. Factors associated with COVID-19-related death in people with rheumatic diseases: results from the COVID-19 Global Rheumatology Alliance physician-reported registry. *Ann Rheum Dis*. 2021;80(7):930–942.

64. Yasmin F, Najeeb H, Naeem U, et al. Adverse events following COVID-19 mRNA vaccines: a systematic review of cardiovascular complication, thrombosis, and thrombocytopenia. *Immun Inflamm Dis*. 2023;11(3):e807.

65. Fazlollahi A, Zahmatyar M, Noori M, et al. Cardiac complications following mRNA COVID-19 vaccines: a systematic review of case reports and case series. *Rev Med Virol*. 2022;32(4):e2318.

66. Montgomery J, Ryan M, Engler R, et al. Myocarditis following immunization with mRNA COVID-19 vaccines in members of the US military. *JAMA Cardiol*. 2021;6(10):1202–1206.

67. Mehta P, Gasparyan AY, Zimba O, et al. Systemic lupus erythematosus in the light of the COVID-19 pandemic: infection, vaccination, and impact on disease management. *Clin Rheumatol*. 2022;41(9):2893–2910.

68. Eryavuz Onmaz D, Tezcan D, Abusoglu S, et al. Effects of hydroxychloroquine and its metabolites in patients with connective tissue diseases. *Inflammopharmacology*. 2021;29(6):1795–1805.

69. Leong DP, Lenihan DJ. Clinical practice guidelines in cardio-oncology. *Heart Fail Clin*. 2022;18(3):489–501.

70. Hsu C-Y, Lin Y-S, Su Y-J, et al. Effect of long-term hydroxychloroquine on vascular events in patients with systemic lupus erythematosus: a database prospective cohort study. *Rheumatology*. 2017;56:2212–2221.

71. Arachchillage DJ, Laffan M, Pericleous C. Hydroxychloroquine as an immunomodulatory and antithrombotic treatment in antiphospholipid syndrome. *Int J Mol Sci*. 2023 Jan;24(2):1331.

72. Morel N, Bonjour M, Le Guern V, et al. Colchicine: a simple and effective treatment for pericarditis in systemic lupus erythematosus? A report of 10 cases. *Lupus.* 2015;24(14):1479–1485.

73. Cavalli G, Colafrancesco S, Emmi G, et al. Interleukin 1α: a comprehensive review on the role of IL-1α in the pathogenesis and treatment of autoimmune and inflammatory diseases. *Autoimmun Rev.* 2021;20(3):102763.

74. Urowitz MB, Aranow C, Asukai Y, et al. Impact of belimumab on organ damage in systemic lupus erythematosus. *Arthritis Care Res (Hoboken).* 2022;74(11):1822–1828.

75. Kalunian KC, Furie R, Morand EF, et al. A randomized, placebo-controlled phase III extension trial of the long-term safety and tolerability of anifrolumab in active systemic lupus erythematosus. *Arthritis Rheumatol.* 2023;75(2):253–265.

76. Grundy SM, Pasternak R, Greenland P, Smith S Jr, Fuster V. Assessment of cardiovascular risk by use of multiple-risk-factor assessment equations: a statement for healthcare professionals from the American Heart Association and the American College of Cardiology. *Circulation.* 1999 Sep 28;100(13):1481–92.

8

Sjogren's syndrome

NASAM ALFRAJI AND LOOMEE DOO

INTRODUCTION

Primary Sjogren's syndrome (pSS) is one of the most common rheumatic diseases, mainly affecting Caucasian middle-aged individuals (1). It is prevalent in 0.05–4.8% of the general population worldwide with a higher incidence among females, outnumbering males at a ratio of 9:1 (1,2). Approximately one-third of pSS patients exhibit extra glandular manifestations (3). Cardiovascular involvement, although an infrequent manifestation, holds significant implications as it is a leading cause of morbidity and mortality in individuals with Sjogren's syndrome. Reported cardiac complications include pericarditis, myocarditis, and, more frequently, congenital heart block (3).

While studies have shown increased traditional cardiac risk factors, such as hypertension, hypertriglyceridemia, and metabolic syndrome, in a minority of patients with pSS, the overall understanding remains limited (3,4). In one cohort study, patients with pSS demonstrated higher rates of cardiovascular disease (61.6% vs. 29.7%; p value <0.05) compared to controls (5). An Italian study observed a higher prevalence of myocardial infarction in patients with pSS compared to control subjects (1.0% vs. 0.4%, p value =0.002) (6). Similarly, a recent meta-analysis reported a higher rate of coronary disease and heart failure (RR 1.34, CI 1.06–1.38, RR 2.54, CI 1.30–4.97, respectively) in pSS patients (7). This study also identified extra glandular involvement as an independent risk factor associated with increased cardiovascular events (5). Additionally, other factors such as purpura, leukopenia, hypocomplementemia,

cryoglobulinemia, and longer disease duration have been associated with increased cardiovascular risk in individuals with pSS (1).

PATHOGENESIS

The primary pathogenic process in pSS involves inflammatory infiltration of exocrine glandular tissue. The glandular infiltrate predominantly consists of T and B lymphocytes and, to a lesser extent, macrophages, plasmacytoid dendritic cells, and natural-killer cells (6). Despite limited research on cardiovascular risk in patients with Sjogren's syndrome, various pathogenic mechanisms have been proposed, including immunological, thrombotic, and pro-atherogenic mechanisms, antibody-mediated endothelial dysfunction, neutrophil cellular activation, and pro-inflammatory cytokines (1).

The upregulation of B and T lymphocytes in pSS has been shown to increase cytokine production such as interleukin (IL)-1β, and other cytokines, leading to further inflammation and a pro-atherogenic response. Additionally, elevated levels of c-reactive protein (CRP) and IL-6 have been identified as independent factors associated with cardiovascular disease in patients with pSS (1).

Immune system dysfunction and the presence of anti-SSA/Ro and anti-SSB/La have been correlated with endothelial damage, an increased intima-media thickness (IMT), and higher risk of cardiovascular events, as summarized in Figure 8.1. Additionally, patients with Sjogren's syndrome have higher endothelial progenitor cells in early disease, which

DOI: 10.1201/9781003386711-8

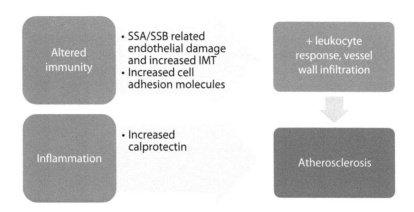

Figure 8.1 Pathogenesis of subclinical atherosclerosis in Sjogren's syndrome.

contribute to repair mechanisms. However, an increase in circulating endothelial microparticles, a marker of damage, has been observed in later stages of the disease, suggesting a decline in repair processes as the disease progresses, thus contributing to accelerated atherosclerosis (3,8).

Some studies in 2004 have reported a form of neutrophil cellular death known as neutrophil extracellular traps (NETs), which might be associated with the development of autoimmune diseases such as pSS. The formation of NETs can be pro-atherogenic and contribute to the progression of cardiovascular diseases in patients with pSS (1).

Antibody-mediated damage has been associated with the development of other cardiac manifestations such as autoimmune congenital heart block in pregnancies exposed to anti-SS antibodies. Anti-SSA/Ro and anti-SSB/La antibodies have a main pathogenic role in congenital heart block along with other risk factors. Anti-Ro52 antibodies, in particular, bind specifically to fetal cardiac cells, leading to apoptosis, inflammatory reactions, and eventually, permanent damage to the AV node, resulting in higher degrees of heart block (1).

CARDIOVASCULAR DISEASE MANIFESTATIONS

Pericarditis

Although overt symptomatic heart disease is rare in Sjogren's syndrome, several studies have shown frequent pericardial diseases in these patients, which were mostly asymptomatic (4). Generally, pericarditis can present with classical symptoms such as sharp, midsternal chest pain upon deep inspiration, shortness of breath while lying supine, palpitations, and low-grade fever. However, asymptomatic pericardial effusions can be another presentation as well (9). In one echocardiographic study, evidence of present or previous pericarditis was observed in 9 out of 27 (33%) pSS patients (10). In another larger study, an echogenic pericardium was revealed in 21 (33%) of 64 pSS patients without any reported clinical symptoms (11). Additionally, a new diagnosis of Sjogren's syndrome was reported in 4 of 61 patients with symptomatic recurrent pericarditis, where pericardial disease was the primary clinical manifestation of their systemic disease in an Italian study (12). Concurrently, a more recent study identified pericardial effusion in 9 of 107 patients with pSS, though this was also associated with concomitant cryoglobulinemia and primary biliary cirrhosis (13).

One of the treatment options of recurrent pericarditis is oral prednisone equivalent dosed at 0.3–0.5 mg/kg/day tapered over two to four weeks. More resistant cases can be treated with steroid-sparing agents such as oral azathioprine at 1–2 mg/kg/day divided into twice-daily dosing, oral or subcutaneous methotrexate up to 20 mg weekly, and oral leflunomide up to 20 mg daily (9).

Myocarditis

Cases of autoimmune myocarditis secondary to pSS have been rarely reported in the literature (4). The diagnosis of myocarditis with pSS in these cases was established after excluding other potential causes. Clinical manifestations are variable, ranging from clinically silent myocarditis to symptoms of congestive heart failure (14,15). Subclinical myocardial involvement can be detected through advanced cardiac imaging techniques such as speckle-tracking echocardiography or cardiac magnetic resonance. However, screening is not recommended in asymptomatic patients without clinical cardiac or ECG abnormalities (1). Autoimmune myocarditis in pSS patients may be associated with systemic visceral vasculitis or inflammatory infiltration of the myocardium (16). Fortunately, most cases respond to corticosteroids and immunosuppressive agents in acute myocarditis in pSS patients (4).

Cardiomyopathy

Given the rarity of this clinical presentation, few reports have discussed cardiomyopathy related to pSS after excluding other etiologies, including ischemic heart disease and infections (17). Patients with cardiomyopathy can present with Sjogren's-related congestive heart failure or as severe as cardiogenic shock (17). There is insufficient data regarding diagnostic criteria or standard therapy for autoimmune cardiomyopathy in pSS (17). However, a few case studies have reported new onset systolic dysfunction in Sjogren's patients who exhibited increased late gadolinium enhancement on cardiac MRI, suggestive of autoimmune process (17,18). Most cases were treated with corticosteroids, along with standard heart failure medication therapy (17). A number of reports have shown promising results with near-to-complete normalization of their cardiac function after a few months of corticosteroids and immunosuppressive therapy (17).

Conduction abnormalities

Autoimmune congenital heart block represents a complication seen in pregnancies exposed to anti-SSA/Ro and/or anti-SSB/La antibodies (anti-SS antibodies). This condition is primarily mediated by the transplacental passage, specifically, of anti-Ro 52 and anti-Ro 60 antibodies to the neonatal cardiac conduction tissue (19). The prevalence of congenital heart block in neonates exposed to anti-SS antibodies during gestation is 1–2% or higher in women with active underlying connective tissue disease and high antibody titers (19). This incidence can increase to 16–18% in cases with prior affected fetuses. The diagnosis of autoimmune congenital heart block can be challenging and it carries high mortality rate, ranging from 12 to 43%. Therefore, serial echocardiogram screening starting as early as 16th week is recommended in anti-Ro-exposed pregnancies (19).

While the cardiac tissue of adults appears to be resistant to the damaging impact of SSA/SSB antibodies, several case reports have revealed an association between these antibodies and heart block in adults as well (20,21). A study published in 2009 showed the co-occurrence of first-degree heart degree block and anti-SSB in patients with pSS (21).

Valvular disease

Valvular disease is uncommon in Sjogren's syndrome, but a few case reports have suggested a potential correlation. A 1984 case report found a patient with a history of chronic Sjogren's disease to have developed aortic and mitral valve stenosis on echocardiogram, with no other comorbidities. It is thought to be caused by chronic inflammation from lymphocyte-mediated valvular destruction. A 2008 study with 109 pSS patients matched to 112 controls found that, though mild, pSS patients had increased cases of mitral, aortic, and tricuspid valve regurgitation on echocardiogram compared to their counterparts (13).

Vasculitis

Vasculitis is a common extraglandular manifestation in pSS that appears early in the disease process. Occasionally, it is the presenting symptom of pSS and affects approximately 15% of this distinct population. In the 2008 GEMESS study, one of the largest cohort studies on pSS, 91 of the 1010 recruited patients were found to have vasculitis. Patients with long-term disease (>10 years) were more likely to develop vasculitis (21).

In another study involving 558 Sjogren's syndrome patients, 51 were found to have cutaneous vasculitis. Of these 51 patients, 14 had type II cryoglobulinemic vasculitis without prior Hepatitis C infection, while 11 had urticarial vasculitis. The remaining 26 patients presented with nonpalpable purpura without evidence of cryoglobulinemia (22). Among the vasculitides, cryoglobulinemic vasculitis is most commonly associated with pSS.

Vasculitis associated with Sjogren's syndrome, however, is not limited to small vessels. A 1987 study found 9 out of 70 patients had vasculitis with a few found to have necrotizing vasculitis in medium vessels. This manifestation may sometimes be confused with polyarteritis nodosa; however, it differs in that it does not present with aneurysms (23). Few case reports have also noted cerebral large vessel vasculitis involvement with pSS, seen by diffuse-weighted MRI, demonstrating homogeneous concentric thickening without positive nor negative remodeling, which is characteristic of vasculitis. Unfortunately, the findings lacked histopathologic evidence for confirmation (24).

Vasculitis associated with Sjogren's syndrome has been found to have a fourfold increased risk for B-cell lymphoma and increased morbidity, particularly with extraglandular involvement such as cardiomyopathy. The Vassiliou study found that pSS patients with palpable purpura had increased risk of cardiac valvular disease. Hence, timely identification and treatment of vasculitis with pSS are essential for overall increased patient survival and lifespan (25).

Cardiovascular disease and accelerated atherosclerosis

As is often found in autoimmune diseases, patients with pSS have an increased risk of cardiovascular disease due to the systemic impact of immune dysregulation. pSS has a known increased risk of major adverse cardiac events, including both coronary events and cerebrovascular events (6). A systematic review and meta-analysis found an increased risk of heart failure associated with pSS. However, the study did not find significantly increased risk of cardiovascular mortality among pSS patients compared to the general population (7).

The increased production of cytokines IL-1β, IL-6, as well as CRP in pSS is believed to contribute to the promotion of atherosclerosis (6). A meta-analysis conducted by Yong and colleagues aimed to determine the risk of subclinical atherosclerosis among pSS patients and their controls. Multiple studies have utilized two measures, IMT and pulse wave velocity (PWV), to determine arterial stiffness. Higher values of these measures are thought to correlate with subclinical atherosclerosis. Among eight eligible studies, three utilized PWV and five employed IMT measures. These studies demonstrated a statistically significant increase in carotid IMT (MD = 0.08 mm; 95% CI 0.04–0.11; p value < 0.01; I2 = 72%) and PWV (MD = 1.30 m/s; 95% CI 0.48–2.12; p value = 0.002; I2 = 85%) in pSS patients compared to controls. This suggests that pSS is associated with a higher risk of subclinical atherosclerosis (26). However, the study had limitations, including a lack of clarity in determining disease duration, severity, and specific antibody associations that might place pSS patients at a higher risk for accelerated atherosclerosis. While it is theoretically believed that long disease duration is associated with higher risk of atherosclerosis, there has been no direct correlation between increased risk of atherosclerosis and increased pSS disease activity or duration (27). Furthermore, typical medications used to treat pSS, such as corticosteroids (HR=1.45, 1.07–1.97) and non-steroidal anti-inflammatory drugs (HR=1.31, 1.05–1.65), have been found to increase the risk of coronary artery disease (28). Large-scale studies are needed to further elucidate the direct association of accelerated atherosclerosis to pSS.

Treatment considerations

Treatment options for cardiac manifestations associated with pSS vary. However, the initial treatment regimen generally consists of corticosteroid therapy that can most rapidly decrease inflammation.

For pericarditis and myocarditis, treatment consists of prednisone as well as steroid-sparing agents like azathioprine, leflunomide, and methotrexate (4,9). Cardiomyopathy from pSS, in addition to steroids, would require heart failure therapy including diuretics, beta blockers as seen in other forms of cardiomyopathy. Some patients responded to intravenous cyclophosphamide as an immunosuppressive agent as well (16). However, due to significant side effects, including increased risk for bladder cancer, cyclophosphamide is often considered a second or third treatment option.

In cases of autoimmune congenital conduction abnormalities, early measures are essential, including fetal screening with weekly echocardiograms starting from the 16th week of pregnancy to at least the 24th week in females with known positive anti-SSA/Ro and anti-SSB/La antibodies or previous history of an affected pregnancy (19). Close monitoring and early detection of cardiac abnormalities play a key role in the prevention and treatment of neonatal cardiac disease. Several preventive and treatment options include glucocorticoids, intravenous immunoglobulin (IVIG), and hydroxychloroquine.

Hydroxychloroquine, when administered from the tenth week of gestation, is particularly effective in preventing CHB in high-risk pregnancies, whereas the use of IVIG and/or fluorinated steroids has not demonstrated similar efficacy throughout pregnancy (19). Complete congenital heart block is considered permanent; therefore, early delivery and lifelong pacemaker implantation are required in such cases (4).

Valvular disease may require surgical intervention for severe cases of regurgitation, but generally, no additional intervention is needed for mild cases. Vasculitis treatment generally depends on the type of vasculitis as well as the extent of disease. For cryoglobulinemic vasculitis commonly seen in pSS, rituximab combined with corticosteroids is the treatment of choice. Alternative options include steroid-sparing agents such as cyclophosphamide, azathioprine, and methotrexate. Refractory cases can also consider mycophenolate mofetil, tumor necrosis factor (TNF) inhibitors, and belimumab (25).

For cardiovascular disease and accelerated atherosclerosis, it is imperative that preventative measures are taken to decrease the risk of these sequelae. Lipid control with cholesterol-lowering medications as well as maintaining good control of pre-existing hypertension and diabetes is essential. Wu and colleagues found that pSS patients have higher incidences of coronary artery disease, hyperlipidemia, and diabetes (28). Thus, providers must be more vigilant in screening and treating these comorbidities for the improvement of overall patient survival.

REFERENCES

1. Casian M, Jurcut C, Dima A, et al. Cardiovascular disease in primary Sjögren's syndrome: raising clinicians' awareness. Front Immunol. 2022 Jun 9;13:865373.

2. Helmick CG, Felson DT, Lawrence RC, et al. Estimates of the prevalence of arthritis and other rheumatic conditions in the United States: Part I. Arthritis Rheum. 2008 Jan;58(1):15–25.

3. Atzeni F, Gozza F, Cafaro G, et al. Cardiovascular involvement in Sjögren's syndrome. Front Immunol. 2022 May 6;13:879516.

4. Melissaropoulos K, Bogdanos D, Dimitroulas T, et al. Primary Sjögren's syndrome and cardiovascular disease. Curr Vasc Pharmacol. 2020;18(5):447–54.

5. Cai X, Luo J, Wei T, et al. Risk of cardiovascular involvement in patients with primary Sjögren's syndrome: a large-scale cross-sectional cohort study. Acta Reumatol Port. 2019 Jan–Mar;44(1):71–7.

6. Bartoloni E, Baldini C, Schillaci G, et al. Cardiovascular disease risk burden in primary Sjögren's syndrome: results of a population-based multicentre cohort study. J Intern Med. 2015 Aug;278(2):185–92.

7. Beltai A, Barnetche T, Daien C, et al. Cardiovascular morbidity and mortality in primary Sjögren's syndrome: a systematic review and meta-analysis. Arthritis Care Res. 2020 Jan;72(1):131–9.

8. Berardicurti O, Ruscitti P, Cipriani P, et al. Cardiovascular disease in primary Sjögren's syndrome. Rev Recent Clin Trials. 2018;13(3):164–9.

9. Barkhodari A, Yao Q. Pericarditis in systemic rheumatologic diseases. Curr Cardiol Rep. 2020;22(11):1–12.

10. Rantapää-Dahlqvist S, Backman C, Sandgren H, et al. Echocardiographic findings in patients with primary Sjögren's syndrome. Clin Rheumatol. 1993;12(2):214–8.

11. Gyöngyösi M, Pokorny G, Jambrik Z, Kovács L, Kovács A, Makula E, et al. Cardiac manifestations in primary Sjögren's syndrome. Ann Rheum Dis. 1996 Jul;55(7):450–4.

12. Brucato A, Brambilla G, Moreo A, et al. Long-term outcomes in difficult-to-treat patients with recurrent pericarditis. Am J Cardiol. 2006 Jul 15;98(2):267–71.

13. Vassiliou VA, Moyssakis I, Boki KA, et al. Is the heart affected in primary Sjögren's syndrome? An echocardiographic study. Clin Exp Rheumatol. 2008;26(1):109–12.

14. Levin MD, Zoet-Nugteren SK, Markusse HM. Myocarditis and primary Sjogren's syndrome. Lancet. 1999 Jul 10;354(9173):128–9.

15. Watanabe T, Takahashi Y, Hirabayashi K, et al. Acute fulminant myocarditis in a patient with primary Sjögren's syndrome. Scand J Rheumatol. 2018;48(2):164–5.

16. Golan TD, Keren D, Elias N, et al. Grand rounds from international lupus centres severe reversible cardiomyopathy associated with systemic vasculitis in primary Sjögren's syndrome. Lupus. 1997;6(6):505–8.

17. Al Turk Y, Lemor A, Fayed M, Kim H. Sjögren-related cardiomyopathy presenting with cardiogenic shock. BMJ Case Rep. 2021;14(10):e244451.

18. Llanos-Chea F, Velasquez A, De Cicco I, et al. Acute heart failure due to anti-RO/SSA and anti-LA/SSB myocarditis in primary Sjogren syndrome. J Am Coll Cardiol. 2016;67(13S):1025.

19. De Carolis S, Garufi C, Garufi E, et al. Autoimmune congenital heart block: a review of biomarkers and management of pregnancy. Front Pediatr. 2020;8:607515.

20. Lee LA, Pickrell MB, Reichlin M. Development of complete heart block in an adult patient with Sjögren's syndrome and anti-Ro/SS-A autoantibodies. Arthritis Rheum. 1996;39(8):1427–9.

21. Ramos-Casals M, Solans R, Rosas J, et al. Primary Sjögren syndrome in Spain: clinical and immunologic expression in 1010 patients. Medicine. 2008;87(4):210–9.

22. Ramos-Casals M, Anaya JM, García-Carrasco M, et al. Cutaneous vasculitis in primary Sjögren syndrome: classification and clinical significance of 52 patients. Medicine. 2004;83(2):96–106.

23. Tsokos M, Lazarou SA, Moutsopoulos HM. Vasculitis in primary Sjögren's syndrome. Histologic classification and clinical presentation. Am J Clin Pathol. 1987;88(1):26–31.

24. Unnikrishnan G, Hiremath N, Chandrasekharan K, et al. Cerebral large-vessel vasculitis in Sjogren's syndrome: utility of high-Resolution magnetic resonance vessel wall imaging. J Clin Neurol. 2018;14(4):588–90.

25. Argyropoulou OD, Tzioufas AG. Common and rare forms of vasculitis associated with Sjögren's syndrome. Curr Opin Rheumatol. 2020;32(1):21–8.

26. Yong WC, Sanguankeo A, Upala S. Association between primary Sjogren's syndrome, arterial stiffness, and subclinical atherosclerosis: a systematic review and meta-analysis. Clin Rheumatol. 2019;38(2):447–55.

27. Berger M, Fesler P, Roubille C. Arterial stiffness, the hidden face of cardiovascular risk in autoimmune and chronic inflammatory rheumatic diseases. Autoimmun Rev. 2021;20(9):102891.

28. Wu XF, Huang JY, Chiou JY, et al. Increased risk of coronary heart disease among patients with primary Sjögren's syndrome: a nationwide population-based cohort study. Sci Rep. 2018;8(1):2209.

9

Systemic sclerosis

NOELLE A. ROLLE, MUHAMMAD UMAIR JAVAID, AND RYAN MASSAY

INTRODUCTION

The current terminology used to describe sclero-derma highlights a culmination of progressive insights in our understanding of the disease. The word 'scleroderma' first appeared in medical litera-ture in 1836 when it was used by the Italian phy-sician Giovambattista Fantonetti to describe the skin changes in one of his patients, though it was introduced into medical terminology by French physician Elie Gintrac (1). The word is a combi-nation of the Greek words 'skleros' and 'derma,' translating to 'hard skin,' a finding considered to be one of the hallmark features of the disease. The significance of this characteristic skin involve-ment is evident in historical accounts, with some attributing the earliest description of the disease to Hippocrates, who reported on an Athenian indi-vidual whose skin was so tight that 'it was not pos-sible to raise it in folds' (2). While the first detailed description is often credited to Carlo Curzio, who described scleroderma-like skin involvement in a young girl in Naples in 1753, contemporary evalua-tion of Curzio's case have led many to believe that it may have represented a scleroderma mimic known as scleredema (3). This diagnostic discrepancy exemplifies the narrow and predominant focus placed on cutaneous involvement in our early understanding of this disease.

The term 'scleroderma' belies many of its more sinister manifestations. Recognition of its multisys-tem involvement was first described by Sir William Osler in 1862, who commented on 'the remarkable

vasomotor disturbances' of patients who were 'apt to succumb to pulmonary complaints or nephritis' (4). Despite this critical, albeit cursory, observa-tion, the systemic nature of the disease was only truly appreciated much later. The initial work by Heine in 1926, followed by a case series by Weiss and Warren in 1943, further expanded the list of organ involvement by outlining a variety of car-diac manifestations associated with scleroderma (5). This shifting paradigm in scleroderma resulted in a proposal by Robert Goetz in 1945 to use the term 'progressive systemic sclerosis,' reflecting a more modern and accurate understanding of the disease (6,7). This terminology has become part of the current nomenclature, classifying scleroderma into a localized form largely limited to the skin (subtypes of morphea and linear scleroderma) and the systemic form, referred to as systemic sclerosis (SSc), characterized by organ involvement. SSc can be further categorized based on the extent of skin involvement into diffuse cutaneous (DSSc), limited cutaneous (LSSc), and SSc sine scleroderma, each with varying degrees of severity and predilection for organ involvement.

EPIDEMIOLOGY

Although our understanding of SSc as a proto-typical systemic disease is firmly established, our comprehension of its role in one of its key target organs – the heart – remains mostly in its infancy. In fact, simply defining the epidemiology of car-diac involvement in scleroderma has proven to be

DOI: 10.1201/9781003386711-9

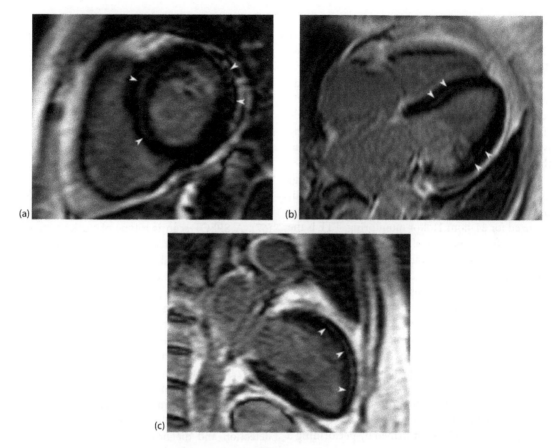

Figure 9.2 Representative delayed enhanced magnetic resonance images in a patient with systemic sclerosis. (a) Short-axis view showing linear mid-wall enhancement (arrowheads) at mid-cavity segments of the interventricular septum. (b) Four-chamber plane showing linear mid-wall enhancement (arrowheads) at basal and mid-cavity segments of the left ventricular (LV) freewall, as well as at the mid-cavity segment of the interventricular septum. (c) Long-axis view showing extensive linear mid-wall enhancement (arrowheads) of the LV anterior wall. (From ref. [36]).

TREATMENT CONSIDERATIONS

To date, there are no official guidelines on the management or trials to assess specific medications or procedures in the management of SSc-related heart disease. Therefore, most of the treatment strategies outlined in Table 9.2 are based on approaches used with non-SSc patients.

The impact of medications on SSc and CVD

Arrhythmias. Methotrexate may induce right bundle branch block and ventricular arrhythmias in rare instances (49). Beta-blocker use may aggravate Raynauds' Disease (RD). Nifedipine is used for RD but has been associated with tachycardia. Calcium channel blockers (CCBs) have been shown to be protective of LV ejection fraction. Consider verapamil as the CCB for atrial and intranodal tachycardia. Hydroxychloroquine is safer than chloroquine regarding conduction disorders. Domperidone is used as a prokinetic for SSc-related gastrointestinal complications but can increase the risk of serious ventricular arrhythmias and sudden cardiac death. Amiodarone is an effective anti-arrhythmic drug but may worsen pulmonary fibrosis.

Pericardial disease. Moderate asymptomatic pericardial effusion may predict occurrence of early or future renal crisis. Monitor kidneys while on NSAIDs for acute pericarditis.

particularly difficult. One of the key impediments in this objective has been the asymptomatic nature of cardiac disease, which may be noted in upward of 70% of patients with cardiac involvement (8).

In addition, primary cardiac disease can result in a wide variety of manifestations that require a heightened level of vigilance for diagnosis. Coupled with these challenges is the reality that our diagnostic devices vary greatly in their individual sensitivities, so clinical suspicion must remain high. Early attempts at investigating the extent of cardiac disease in patients with SSc revealed that up to 80%–90% had notable inflammatory, fibrotic, or vasculopathic changes in the myocardium on autopsy (9). Unfortunately, neither symptoms nor findings from electrocardiograms (ECGs) or echocardiograms (ECHO) reliably predicted the presence of cardiac fibrosis on autopsy (10). It should be noted, however, that although evaluation through autopsy allows for detection of definitive involvement, it is obviously biased toward detection in patients with the highest burden of disease given their mortality. With these previously mentioned limitations in mind, the overall clinical prevalence of cardiac disease is estimated to be around 15%–35% (8).

The significance of cardiac disease in SSc is underscored by its substantial contribution to mortality, with estimates of up to 70% mortality at 5 years in patients with clinical cardiac disease (11). According to the 2010 EUSTAR database, the majority of deaths in SSc, around 33%, were secondary to pulmonary causes; however, death from cardiac disease was tied with death from pulmonary arterial hypertension (PAH) at 14% for the second most common cause of death overall (12).

PATHOPHYSIOLOGY

The mechanisms behind cardiovascular manifestations of SSc are consistent with the underlying pathophysiology of SSc in other organs. The classic triad of SSc includes immune system activation, microvascular dysfunction, and tissue fibrosis. Myocardial dysfunction, for example, appears to begin with microvascular changes and collagen overproduction that leads to concentric intimal hyperplasia of the intramural arteries. Subsequently, this process results in abnormal perfusion, ischemia, and fibrinoid necrosis, manifesting

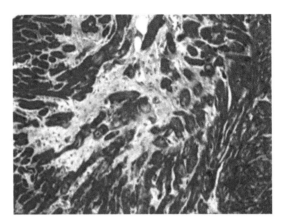

Figure 9.1 Patchy myocardial fibrosis. (From ref. [22].)

with the pathologic hallmark of patchy myocardial fibrosis, as seen in Figure 9.1 (5). This same pathologic mechanism of fibrosis can be responsible for the development of conduction abnormalities, cardiomyopathy, and pericardial and valvular disease.

The existence of a cardiac Raynaud phenomenon (RP) has also been reported to be another possible mechanism of disease in SSc. In a review of sclerodermic cardiomyopathy, Giucă and colleagues cited multiple studies demonstrating cardiac perfusion abnormalities on positron emission tomography (PET), single photon emission tomography (SPECT), and cardiac magnetic resonance (CMR) after cold provocation (13). This finding has been associated with the development of left ventricle contractile dysfunction. In contrast to peripheral RP, myocardial RP appears to show only limited luminal narrowing of the smaller arteries and arterioles (14). The vascular spasms associated with myocardial RP can result in repeated ischemia-reperfusion injuries that eventually lead to the development of contraction band necrosis and fibrosis (13, 15). Although contraction band necrosis is a histologic marker for cardiac involvement, it is also classically seen in atherosclerotic disease. However, key features distinguishing the fibrosis seen in scleroderma and atherosclerotic ischemia are the typical sparing of subendocardial tissue in atherosclerosis and the lack of hemosiderin deposits in SSc (14).

In essence, a great many details surrounding the nature of cardiac disease in SSc remain in need of further investigation. However, there is little doubt that the involvement of the heart in SSc is an important manifestation of the disease.

CARDIOVASCULAR DISEASE MANIFESTATIONS

Patients with cardiac involvement will present with symptoms and signs similar to those of the general population. These include chest pain (exertional, positional, pleuritic, or at rest), dyspnea (exertional, at rest, paroxysmal nocturnal), nocturnal cough, palpitations, orthopnea, and pre-syncopal or syncopal events. Cardiac manifestations may occur early (within the first 5 years) (16) or late in the disease course (17) with onset being defined as the first non-Raynaud symptom (16). Table 9.1 outlines the manifestations, which are varied and most often subclinical initially (16).

Risk factors for cardiac involvement include severity of nailfold capillaroscopy (16,17) and antibody subtype (anti-topoisomerase, anti-Ku, anti-U3 RNP, ant histone, anti-ribonucleic acid [RNA] polymerase [I, II, III] antibodies) (13). RNA polymerase 3 is associated with cor-pulmonale with minimal pulmonary fibrosis, suggesting that the

PAH as a result of vasculopathy (18). In one study, the Modified Rodnan Skin Score, used to assess severity of skin disease, was associated with higher heart rate variability and lower RV ejection fraction (19). Cardiac disease frequency in SSc is also thought to increase as nailfold capillaroscopy patterns progress (17).

Pericardial disease

Symptomatic pericarditis is estimated to occur in 7%–20% of patients (20,21), but the incidence may be as high as 72%. In an autopsy series conducted on 44 patients with SSc, chronic pericarditis was detected in 31 cases and was more frequent than myocardial fibrosis (15/44) (20). This suggests that pericardial involvement is mostly asymptomatic. Additional pericardial manifestations include fibrinous pericarditis, constrictive pericarditis, and pericardial adhesions. Fibrosis of the myocardium and pericardium can predispose to restrictive and constrictive cardiomyopathy, respectively (22). Pericardial effusions are usually small, asymptomatic, and exudative. Transudative effusions in the setting of right heart failure are more responsive to diuretics. Large pericardial effusions are a risk factor for the development of scleroderma renal crisis (5).

Atherosclerosis

Cardiovascular disease (CVD), the leading cause of mortality and a major contributor to morbidity globally, is strongly influenced by atherosclerosis (23). The risk of atherosclerosis is increased in systemic autoimmune diseases, including rheumatoid arthritis (RA), systemic lupus erythematosus (SLE), and systemic vasculitis. This has led to the creation of the term 'accelerated atherosclerosis', which is postulated to be a phenomenon occurring in patients with systemic autoimmune diseases due to the interaction of traditional and non-traditional risk factors, including an inflammatory state, lipid oxidation, anti-oxidized LDL autoantibody production, endothelial dysfunction, glucocorticoid use, and smoking (24). Although the presence of anti-cardiolipin and β2-glycoprotein I antibodies is rare in SSc, either one may be implicated in the mechanism of CVD in SSc, with the latter presenting as an independent predictor of mortality in one study (25).

Table 9.1 Cardiac manifestations of SSc

Pericardial	Acute pericarditis, chronic pericarditis, pericardial fibrosis, pericardial effusion, tamponade
Myocardial	Myocardial fibrosis, ventricular diastolic dysfunction, ventricular systolic dysfunction, myocarditis
Conduction system disease	Autonomic dysfunction, heart block, supraventricular dysrhythmia, ventricular dysrhythmia
Vascular	Mural fibrosis, intimal proliferation, platelet-fibrin clotting

Accelerated atherosclerosis also occurs in SSc due, in part, to calcification, vasculopathy, and endothelial wall damage. When compared to healthy controls, the prevalence of coronary atherosclerosis, peripheral vascular disease, and cerebrovascular calcification is higher in SSc (26). These patients have higher rates of subclinical atherosclerosis (27), higher coronary artery calcium scores (28), more coronary plaques, and a four times greater risk of developing carotid plaques (24). It is suggested that extra-coronary calcification may appear earlier or in the absence of coronary artery calcification and maybe a marker of SSc-associated atherosclerosis (29).

Cited risk factors for atherosclerosis in SSc include age, cumulative dose of steroids > 10 g prednisone equivalent (27), and centromere antibody positivity (29,30). Longer disease duration, higher BMI, left ventricular (LV) mass, and LV mass index were also found to correlate with higher coronary artery scores (29).

Importantly, while the rate of subclinical atherosclerosis is similar to RA (31), the outcomes may be worse. Retrospective observational data revealed that hospitalized SSc patients with atherosclerotic CVD had a higher mortality than their RA and SLE counterparts (32).

Vascular disease

Smaller arteries and arterioles are predominantly affected in SSc. Vasospasm of these vessels is thought to play a significant role in the early myocardial abnormalities observed. Angina and myocardial infarction may occur in the absence of significant epicardial arterial disease because of intramural coronary artery involvement. This manifests histologically as concentric intimal hyperplasia with fibrinoid necrosis (5).

Myocardial disease

Microvascular disease, which leads to ischemia-reperfusion injury, subsequent necrosis, eventual fibrosis, and then remodeling, is thought to be the inciting event for the onset of myocardial involvement (33).

The prevalence of myocardial involvement may be up to 45% and is more common in DSSc than LSSc (34). Other risk factors for primary involvement are advanced age, rapid progression of skin

thickening, male gender, duration of disease, digital ulcers, simultaneous renal and muscular impairment, disease activity score, pulmonary fibrosis, PAH (35), duration of Raynauds > 15 years (36), and more severe nailfold capillaroscopy findings (16).

Systolic, with an estimated incidence of 11%–15%, typically occurs as a result of concomitant ischemic or hypertensive heart disease (5). Independent factors for LV dysfunction include male sex, digital ulcers, and myositis. Calcium channel blocker use may have a protective effect against this (37).

SSc-related cardiomyopathy progresses over time and can be detected by speckle-tracking global longitudinal strain (GLS). This parameter is a measure of systolic function and is thought to be more reproducible than the ejection fraction (38). The endocardial layers of the ventricles show the greatest change, as demonstrated in a 2020 SSc study, where decreases in GLS as low as 1% in the right ventricle were shown to significantly increase the risk of PAH (55% increase, p = 0.043), all-cause death, and major cardiovascular events (18% increase p = 0.03) (39). A similar study of 234 SSc patients prospectively assessed changes in cardiac performance and found that progression of LV systolic dysfunction was demonstrated by GLS but not by LV ejection fraction. Individuals at greatest risk for progression were identified as those with proximal muscle weakness, decreased DLCO, and LV diastolic dysfunction (40).

Diastolic dysfunction, which can affect both ventricles, is more common than systolic failure and more common compared to the general population with a prevalence ranging between 15% and 62%. Risk factors include advanced age, systemic hypertension, disease duration, CVD, SSc lung complications, and impaired systolic function, although it may occur in the absence of such comorbidities (41–44). As LV diastolic dysfunction progresses over time, the risk for mortality increases and exceeds that of PAH (45).

Cardiac MRI features of myocardial involvement include late gadolinium enhancement (LGE) in a linear (DSSc) or patchy nodular pattern (LSSc) that spares the subendocardial layers and exhibits a predilection for the basal and mid-cavity segments of the left ventricle. The subendocardial sparing, which deviates from the regional distribution of a single vascular pattern, differentiates it from ischemic cardiomyopathy and myocarditis (46). LGE on cardiac MRI is further associated with a higher prevalence of ECG abnormalities (46). Histologically, reported changes involve diffuse patchy fibrosis with contraction band necrosis, a haphazard lesion distribution unrelated to epicardial coronary stenosis (5), and concentric intimal hypertrophy, all of which are associated with fibrinoid necrosis of intramural coronary arteries (47).

Myocarditis may arise in primary disease (45) but is more commonly part of an overlap syndrome (5,48).

Conduction abnormalities

Dysrhythmias are postulated to account for approximately 6% of SSc-related cardiovascular mortalities (12). Underlying mechanisms that may account for ECG abnormalities include transient oxygen-supply imbalance, myocardial fibrosis, conduction system fibrosis, and autonomic cardiac neuropathy (49,50).

The electrophysiological abnormalities observed in ECGs are extremely varied, ranging from interval prolongation to conduction blockades, tachycardias (atrial and ventricular), and malignant dysrhythmias. These latter rhythms stand as the third most common cause of death in SSc patients, responsible for 5% of mortality (50).

Resting ECG abnormalities, including left bundle branch block and first-degree atrioventricular block, have been found in 19%–52% of patients (51–53). QTc prolongation was found in up to 25% in a cohort of 689 scleroderma patients, 14.6% of whom had no cardiac symptoms (54). Patients with ventricular ectopic beats exceeding 1190 in a 24-hour period are identified as high-risk for life-threatening arrhythmic complications (55). Ventricular dysrhythmias can occur in both early (within 3 years) and late (after 6 years) disease (50), with no significant difference in occurrence of these rhythms between DSSc and LSSc (56).

Right bundle branch block is an independent predictor of mortality in SSc as reported by Draeger and colleagues, whereby the risk of mortality increased 5.3-fold in a cohort of 265 SSc patients with early disease who were prospectively followed for 9 years (53).

Valvular heart disease

Valvular heart disease (VHD) occurs relatively infrequently. Overall, 17% of patients in a cohort of 86, studied between 2010 and 2011, had valvular abnormalities affecting the mitral, aortic, and tricuspid valves in 4%, 8%, and 9% of cases, respectively (51). The latter occurred exclusively in association with pulmonary hypertension. Similarly in a prospective cohort of 570 patients, mitral regurgitation was detected in 6.7%, while 3.3% had aortic stenosis and 2.5% aortic regurgitation (57).

Despite ongoing debates regarding the most common valvular abnormality, various reports suggest that nodular thickening of the mitral and aortic valves, leading to hemodynamically insignificant regurgitation, constitutes the most common lesions. One study even reported a 60% rate of asymptomatic mitral valve prolapse (22,58). However, a retrospective prevalence study of newly diagnosed SSc patients found tricuspid regurgitation, mostly, but not solely, related to PAH to be the most common abnormality (59). The study concluded that patients with SSc have a four-fold increase in the prevalence of moderate/severe VHD at diagnosis compared to non-SSc patients (MR, TR, and PR). Furthermore, there is a four-fold increased risk of developing moderate/severe VHD after diagnosis of SSc. Aortic stenosis had a higher-than-expected prevalence in that study (59).

Endocardial disease

The association between SSc and endocarditis with valvular disease is infrequent (48).

Vasculitis

To date, primary vasculitis has not been described in patients with SSc. The presence thereof suggests an overlap syndrome with other connective tissue diseases such as SLE, ANCA vasculitis, or mixed cryoglobulinemic vasculitis related to Sjogren's Syndrome (5,60,61). Overlaps to ANCA vasculitis seem to be more common with LSSc, manifesting as microscopic polyangiitis with positive myeloperoxidase antibodies (61).

SCREENING

Cardiac involvement in SSc occurs early in the disease process and is asymptomatic. Therefore, screening should occur at diagnosis and include baseline and annual 12-lead ECG, transthoracic echocardiogram (TTE), b-type natriuretic peptide (BNP), and troponin levels. Autoantibody testing is also important as specific antibodies may inform the need for closer cardiac monitoring (8,13).

An ECG (resting and ambulatory monitoring) assists with identification of conduction abnormalities and pericardial disease and can help determine the need for 24-hour Holtor monitoring. TTE is the mainstay for evaluation of cardiac involvement in SSc and can assess various forms of involvement including pericardial, myocardial, and valvular disease, coronary artery disease, and PAH (62).

All patients with SSc, regardless of type and antibody profile, are at risk for developing PAH. There is an increased risk for those with long disease duration, male gender, increased telangiectasias, reduced capillary nailfold density, and anti-centromere antibody positivity. Screening should be done annually and can be accomplished using the DETECT algorithm (63–65). While suggested by TTE, PAH is confirmed by performing a right heart catheterization.

Elevated levels of BNP > 60 pg/mL or N-terminal pro BNP (NT-pro-BNP) > 125 pg/mL suggest possible cardiovascular involvement. In particular, a significant increase in these levels from baseline is suspicious for cardiac involvement or PAH (64,65). Other biomarkers that can be used for screening and diagnosis include troponin I levels (more specific to the myocardium than troponin T), creatinine kinase, and CK-MB, but their roles have not been defined and it's not clear about their utility in detecting early cardiac involvement. They've been shown to be more reliable in evaluating symptomatic or established cardiac involvement. An issue with these markers is that they are not specific for SSc and can be elevated in other SSc manifestations such as ischemic heart disease, PAH, and renal impairment.

DIAGNOSTIC EVALUATION

Additional testing from baseline is directed by symptoms and signs found on history and physical exam as well as indicated in those with abnormal screening tests outlined above. These second-tier testing are also used as pre-evaluation testing for cardiac involvement in patients preparing for hematopoietic stem cell transplantation (HSCT).

One of the latest advancements for evaluating subclinical myocardial dysfunction is to use a two-dimensional speckle-tracking echocardiography (STE) strain analysis, which can be used to evaluate both global and regional LV and RV systolic function (66). STE-derived GLS and global circumferential strain (GCS) are significantly impaired in SSc when compared with healthy controls and these have been associated with ventricular arrhythmias (67). A SPECT scan is a type of nuclear imaging test that can characterize the function and perfusion of the myocardium. Perfusion defects have been noted in patients with both DSSc and LSSc and can be found in patients with normal systolic function. Coronary angiography is utilized to evaluate for coronary artery disease.

Cardiac MRI (CMR) (Figure 9.2) noninvasively assesses cardiac function and performs tissue characterization that avoids the use of radiation and is operator independent. T2-weighted imaging can detect edema, infiltration, ischemia, and focal or diffuse fibrosis of the cardiac muscles for early detection and diagnosis of heart involvement in SSc that cannot be detected with other modalities. LGE is considered the best way to detect myocardial fibrosis. T1-mapping (a measurement of the relaxation time of myocardial tissue) and extracellular volume quantification, which are both found to be significantly higher in patients with SSc than healthy controls, help to quantify diffuse fibrosis and are associated with future ventricular arrhythmic events (68,69). CT, CMR, and LGE can also be used for further evaluation of valvular involvement.

Endomyocardial or biopsies can help distinguish between SSc involvement and other conditions such as sarcoidosis and other causes of myocarditis. A risk of false-negative testing is to be considered due to the patchy nature of myocardial involvement and risk of sampling error. Complications are reported in 1%–3.3% of procedures done. There is no one specific finding on pathology. Rather, findings can range from replacement fibrosis and foci of inflammation to contraction band necrosis, inflammatory infiltrates adjacent to areas of myocyte necrosis or degeneration and lymphocyte infiltrates.

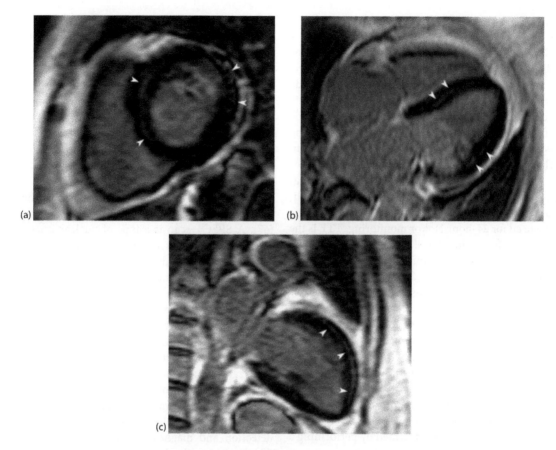

Figure 9.2 Representative delayed enhanced magnetic resonance images in a patient with systemic sclerosis. (a) Short-axis view showing linear mid-wall enhancement (arrowheads) at mid-cavity segments of the interventricular septum. (b) Four-chamber plane showing linear mid-wall enhancement (arrowheads) at basal and mid-cavity segments of the left ventricular (LV) freewall, as well as at the mid-cavity segment of the interventricular septum. (c) Long-axis view showing extensive linear mid-wall enhancement (arrowheads) of the LV anterior wall. (From ref. [36]).

TREATMENT CONSIDERATIONS

To date, there are no official guidelines on the management or trials to assess specific medications or procedures in the management of SSc-related heart disease. Therefore, most of the treatment strategies outlined in Table 9.2 are based on approaches used with non-SSc patients.

The impact of medications on SSc and CVD

Arrhythmias. Methotrexate may induce right bundle branch block and ventricular arrhythmias in rare instances (49). Beta-blocker use may aggravate Raynauds' Disease (RD). Nifedipine is used for RD but has been associated with tachycardia. Calcium channel blockers (CCBs) have been shown to be protective of LV ejection fraction. Consider verapamil as the CCB for atrial and intranodal tachycardia. Hydroxychloroquine is safer than chloroquine regarding conduction disorders. Domperidone is used as a prokinetic for SSc-related gastrointestinal complications but can increase the risk of serious ventricular arrhythmias and sudden cardiac death. Amiodarone is an effective anti-arrhythmic drug but may worsen pulmonary fibrosis.

Pericardial disease. Moderate asymptomatic pericardial effusion may predict occurrence of early or future renal crisis. Monitor kidneys while on NSAIDs for acute pericarditis.

Table 9.2 Treatment strategies for cardiovascular manifestations of SSc

Disease manifestation	Treatment option(s)
Arrhythmias	a. Anti-arrhythmic pharmacotherapy b. Ablation c. Implantable cardioverter defibrillator (ICD) d. Pacemaker
Pericardial effusion	a. NSAIDs b. Cardiac tamponade or constriction – pericardiocentesis or surgical intervention
Myocarditis	a. Corticosteroids b. Azathioprine c. Methotrexate d. Mycophenolate Mofetil e. Cyclophosphamide f. Tocilizumab g. Rituximab
Left ventricular systolic dysfunction	a. Angiotensin-converting enzyme inhibitors b. Beta-blocker c. Diuretics prn d. Cardiac resynchronization therapy e. Heart transplant f. Ivabradine, bosantin, sildenafil, iloprost
Pulmonary arterial hypertension (PAH)	a. Vasoactive therapy
Valvular heart disease	a. Valve replacement

Myocardial disease. Moderate oral doses of corticosteroids have been shown to improve LV systolic function. Balance this with the potential risk of precipitation of scleroderma renal crisis. A retrospective study published in 2023 cited improvement in myocardial involvement as detected by cardiac MRI in patients treated with a myriad of immunosuppressives, including Tociluzimab, Rituximab, and Methotrexate (70).

REFERENCES

1. Gintrac E. Note sur la sclerodermie. Rev Med-Chir (Paris). 1847;2:263–7.
2. Pasero G, Marson P. Hippocrates and rheumatology. Clin Exp Rheumatol. 2004;22(6):687–9.
3. Curzio C. Discussioni anatomico-pratiche di un raro, estravagante morbo cutaneo in una giovane Donna felicemente curato in questo grande Ospedale degl'Incurabili. Napoli: Giovanni di Simone; 1753: 1–13.
4. Osler WMT. Principles and practice of medicine. 10th ed. New York and London: D. Appleton and Company; 1927.
5. Parks JL, Taylor MH, Parks LP, et al. Systemic sclerosis and the heart. Rheum Dis Clin North Am. 2014;40(1):87–102.
6. Goetz RH. Pathology of progressive systemic sclerosis (generalized scleroderma) with special reference to changes in the viscera. Clin Proc S Afr. 1945;4:337–42.
7. Hawk A, English JC 3rd. Localized and systemic scleroderma. Semin Cutan Med Surg. 2001;20(1):27–37.
8. Boueiz A, Mathai SC, Hummers LK, et al. Cardiac complications of systemic sclerosis: recent progress in diagnosis. Curr Opin Rheumatol. 2010;22(6):696–703.
9. D'Angelo WA, Fries JF, Masi AT, et al. Pathologic observations in systemic sclerosis (scleroderma): a study of fifty-eight autopsy cases and fifty-eight matched controls. Am J Med. 1969 Mar 1;46(3):428–40.
10. Sandmeier B, Jager VK, Nagy G, et al. Autopsy versus clinical findings in patients with systemic sclerosis in a case series from patients of the EUSTAR database. Clin Exp Rheumatol. 2015;33(4 Suppl 91):S75–9.
11. Medsger TJ, Masi A. Survival with scleroderma. II. A life-table analysis of clinical and demographic factors in 358 male U.S. veteran patients. J Chronic Dis. 1973;26:647.
12. Tyndall AJ, Bannert B, Vonk M, et al. Causes and risk factors for death in systemic sclerosis: a study from the EULAR Scleroderma Trials and Research (EUSTAR) database. Ann Rheum Dis. 2010;69(10):1809–15.

13. Giucă A, Gegenava T, Mihai CM, et al. Sclerodermic cardiomyopathy – a state-of-the-art review. Diagnostics (Basel). 2022 Mar 9;12(3):669.

14. Champion HC. The heart in scleroderma. Rheum Dis Clin North Am. 2008;34(1):181–90.

15. Belloli L, Carlo-Stella N, Ciocia G, et al. Myocardial involvement in systemic sclerosis. Rheumatology (Oxford). 2008;47(7):1070–2.

16. Cutolo M, Sulli A, Secchi ME, et al. Nailfold capillaroscopy is useful for the diagnosis and follow-up of autoimmune rheumatic diseases. A future tool for the analysis of microvascular heart involvement? Rheumatology (Oxford). 2006;45 (Suppl 4):iv43–6.

17. Caramaschi P, Canestrini S, Martinelli N, et al. Scleroderma patients nailfold video capillaroscopic patterns are associated with disease subset and disease severity. Rheumatology (Oxford). 2007;46(10):1566–9.

18. Murata I, Takenaka K, Shinohara S, et al. Diversity of myocardial involvement in systemic sclerosis: an 8-year study of 95 Japanese patients. Am Heart J. 1998;135(6 Pt 1):960–9.

19. Tadic M, Zlatanovic M, Cuspidi C, et al. Systemic sclerosis impacts right heart and cardiac autonomic nervous system. J Clin Ultrasound. 2018;46(3):188–94.

20. Byers RJ, Marshall DA, Freemont AJ. Pericardial involvement in systemic sclerosis. Ann Rheum Dis. 1997;56(6):393–4.

21. Mavrogeni SI, Bratis K, Karabela G, et al. Cardiovascular magnetic resonance imaging clarifies cardiac pathophysiology in early, asymptomatic diffuse systemic sclerosis. Inflamm Allergy Drug Targets. 2015;14(1):29–36.

22. Hung G, Mercurio V, Hsu S, et al. Progress in understanding, diagnosing, and managing cardiac complications of systemic sclerosis. Curr Rheumatol Rep. 2019;21(12):68.

23. Roth GA, Mensah GA, Johnson CO, et al. Global burden of cardiovascular diseases and risk factors, 1990-2019: update from the GBD 2019 study. J Am Coll Cardiol. 2020;76(25):2982–3021.

24. Sciarra I, Vasile M, Carboni A, et al. Subclinical atherosclerosis in systemic sclerosis: different risk profiles among patients according to clinical manifestations. Int J Rheum Dis. 2021;24(4):502–9.

25. Boin F, Franchini S, Colantuoni E, et al. Independent association of anti-beta(2)-glycoprotein I antibodies with macrovascular disease and mortality in scleroderma patients. Arthritis Rheum. 2009 Aug;60(8):2480–9.

26. Au K, Singh MK, Bodukam V, et al. Atherosclerosis in systemic sclerosis: a systematic review and meta-analysis. Arthritis Rheum. 2011;63(7):2078–90.

27. Vettori S, Maresca L, Cuomo G, et al. Clinical and subclinical atherosclerosis in systemic sclerosis: consequences of previous corticosteroid treatment. Scand J Rheumatol. 2010;39(6):485–9.

28. Khurma V, Meyer C, Park GS, et al. A pilot study of subclinical coronary atherosclerosis in systemic sclerosis: coronary artery calcification in cases and controls. Arthritis Rheum. 2008;59(4):591–7.

29. Afifi N, Khalifa MMM, Al Anany A, et al. Cardiac calcium score in systemic sclerosis. Clin Rheumatol. 2022;41(1):105–14.

30. Nordin A, Jensen-Urstad K, Bjornadal L, et al. Ischemic arterial events and atherosclerosis in patients with systemic sclerosis: a population-based case-control study. Arthritis Res Ther. 2013;15(4):R87.

31. Dimitroulas T, Baniotopoulos P, Pagkopoulou E, et al. Subclinical atherosclerosis in systemic sclerosis and rheumatoid arthritis: a comparative matched-cohort study. Rheumatol Int. 2020;40(12):1997–2004.

32. Dave AJ, Fiorentino D, Lingala B, et al. Atherosclerotic cardiovascular disease in hospitalized patients with systemic sclerosis: higher mortality than patients with lupus and rheumatoid arthritis. Arthritis Care Res (Hoboken). 2014;66(2):323–7.

33. Mok MY, Lau CS. The burden and measurement of cardiovascular disease in systemic sclerosis. Nat Rev Rheumatol. 2010;6:430–4. https://doi.org/10.1038/nrrheum.2010.65.

34. Rodríguez-Reyna TS, Morelos-Guzman M, Hernández-Reyes P, et al. Assessment of myocardial fibrosis and microvascular damage in systemic sclerosis by magnetic resonance imaging and coronary angiotomography. Rheumatology (Oxford). 2015;54(4):647–54.

35. Lambova S. Cardiac manifestations in systemic sclerosis. World J Cardiol. 2014;6(9):993–1005.

36. Tzelepis GE, Kelekis NL, Plastiras SC, et al. Pattern and distribution of myocardial fibrosis in systemic sclerosis: a delayed enhanced magnetic resonance imaging study. Arthritis Rheum. 2007;56(11):3827–36.

37. Meune C, Vignaux O, Kahan A, et al. Heart involvement in systemic sclerosis: evolving concept and diagnostic methodologies. Arch Cardiovasc Dis. 2010;103(1):46–52.

38. Kouris NT, Kostopoulos VS, Psarrou GA, et al. Left ventricular ejection fraction and Global Longitudinal Strain variability between methodology and experience. Echocardiography. 2021;38(4):582–9.

39. Stronati G, Manfredi L, Ferrarini A, et al. Subclinical progression of systemic sclerosis-related cardiomyopathy. Eur J Prev Cardiol. 2020;27(17):1876–86.

40. van Wijngaarden SE, Ben Said-Bouyeri S, Ninaber MK, et al. Progression of left ventricular myocardial dysfunction in systemic sclerosis: a speckle-tracking strain echocardiography study. J Rheumatol. 2019;46(4):405–15.

41. Hinchcliff M, Desai CS, Varga J, Shah SJ. Prevalence, prognosis, and factors associated with left ventricular diastolic dysfunction in systemic sclerosis. Clin Exp Rheumatol. 2012;30:S30–7.

42. Ross L, Patel S, Stevens W, et al. The clinical implications of left ventricular diastolic dysfunction in systemic sclerosis. Clin Exp Rheumatol. 2022;40(10):1986–92.

43. Vemulapalli S, Cohen L, Hsu V. Prevalence and risk factors for left ventricular diastolic dysfunction in a scleroderma cohort. Scand J Rheumatol. 2017;46(4):281–7.

44. Faludi R, Kolto G, Bartos B, Csima G, Czirjak L, Komocsi A. Five-year follow-up of left ventricular diastolic function in systemic sclerosis patients: determinants of mortality and disease progression. Semin Arthritis Rheum. 2014;44(2):220–7.

45. Tennøe AH, Murbræch K, Andreassen JC, et al. Left ventricular diastolic dysfunction predicts mortality in patients with systemic sclerosis. J Am Coll Cardiol. 2018;72(15):1804–13.

46. Di Cesare E, Battisti S, Di Sibio A, et al. Early assessment of sub-clinical cardiac involvement in systemic sclerosis (SSc) using delayed enhancement cardiac magnetic resonance (CE-MRI). Eur J Radiol. 2013;82(6):e268–73.

47. James TN. De subitaneis mortibus. VIII. Coronary arteries and conduction system in scleroderma heart disease. Circulation. 1974;50(4):844–56.

48. Dinser R, Frerix M, Meier FM, Klingel K, Rolf A. Endocardial and myocardial involvement in systemic sclerosis – is there a relevant inflammatory component? Joint Bone Spine. 2013;80(3):320–3.

49. Vacca A, Meune C, Gordon J, et al. Cardiac arrhythmias and conduction defects in systemic sclerosis. Rheumatology (Oxford). 2014;53(7):1172–7.

50. Sebestyen V, Szucs G, Pall D, et al. Electrocardiographic markers for the prediction of ventricular arrhythmias in patients with systemic sclerosis. Rheumatology (Oxford). 2020;59(3):478–86.

51. Roberts NK, Cabeen WR Jr., Moss J, et al. The prevalence of conduction defects and cardiac arrhythmias in progressive systemic sclerosis. Ann Intern Med. 1981;94(1):38–40.

52. Ferri C, Bernini L, Bongiorni MG, et al. Noninvasive evaluation of cardiac dysrhythmias, and their relationship with multisystemic symptoms, in progressive systemic sclerosis patients. Arthritis Rheum. 1985;28(11):1259–66.

53. Draeger HT, Assassi S, Sharif R, et al. Right bundle branch block: a predictor of mortality in early systemic sclerosis. PLOS ONE. 2013;8(10):e78808.

54. Massie C, Hudson M, Tatibouet S, et al. Absence of an association between anti-Ro antibodies and prolonged QTc interval

in systemic sclerosis: a multicenter study of 689 patients. Semin Arthritis Rheum. 2014;44(3):338–44.

55. De Luca G, Bosello SL, Gabrielli FA, et al. Prognostic role of ventricular ectopic beats in systemic sclerosis: a prospective cohort study shows ECG indexes predicting the worse outcome. PLOS ONE. 2016;11(4):e0153012.

56. Muresan L, Oancea I, Mada RO, et al. Relationship between ventricular arrhythmias, conduction disorders, and myocardial fibrosis in patients with systemic sclerosis. J Clin Rheumatol. 2018;24(1):25–33.

57. de Groote P, Gressin V, Hachulla E, et al. Evaluation of cardiac abnormalities by Doppler echocardiography in a large nationwide multicentric cohort of patients with systemic sclerosis. Ann Rheum Dis. 2008;67(1):31–6.

58. Sponga S, Basso C, Ruffatti A, Gerosa G. Systemic sclerosis and aortic valve stenosis: therapeutic implications in two cases of aortic valve replacement. J Cardiovasc Med (Hagerstown). 2009;10(7):560–2.

59. Kurmann RD, El-Am EA, Radwan YA, et al. Increased risk of valvular heart disease in systemic sclerosis: an underrecognized cardiac complication. J Rheumatol. 2021;48(7):1047–52.

60. Saketkoo LA, Distler O. Is there evidence for vasculitis in systemic sclerosis? Curr Rheumatol Rep. 2012;14(6):516–25.

61. Quemeneur T, Mouthon L, Cacoub P, et al. Systemic vasculitis during the course of systemic sclerosis: report of 12 cases and review of the literature. Medicine (Baltimore). 2013;92(1):1–9.

62. Kahan A, Coghlan G, McLaughlin V. Cardiac complications of systemic sclerosis. Rheumatology (Oxford). 2009;48(Suppl 3): iii45–8.

63. Galiè N, McLaughlin VV, Rubin LJ, et al. An overview of the 6th World Symposium on Pulmonary Hypertension. Eur Respir J. 2019;53(1):1802148.

64. Young A, Moles VM, Jaafar S, et al. Performance of the DETECT algorithm for pulmonary hypertension screening in a systemic sclerosis cohort. Arthritis Rheumatol. 2021;73(9):1731–7.

65. Humbert M, Kovacs G, Hoeper MM, et al. 2022 ESC/ERS guidelines for the diagnosis and treatment of pulmonary hypertension. Eur Heart J. 2022;43(38):3618–731.

66. Yiu KH, Schouffoer AA, Marsan NA, et al. Left ventricular dysfunction assessed by speckle-tracking strain analysis in patients with systemic sclerosis: relationship to functional capacity and ventricular arrhythmias. Arthritis Rheum. 2011;63(12):3969–78.

67. Bruni C, Ross L. Cardiac involvement in systemic sclerosis: getting to the heart of the matter. Best Pract Res Clin Rheumatol. 2021;35(3):101668.

68. Ntusi NA, Piechnik SK, Francis JM, et al. Subclinical myocardial inflammation and diffuse fibrosis are common in systemic sclerosis – a clinical study using myocardial T1-mapping and extracellular volume quantification. J Cardiovasc Magn Reson. 2014;16:21.

69. Meloni A, Gargani L, Bruni C, Cavallaro C, Gobbo M, D'Agostino A, D'Angelo G, Martini N, Grigioni F, Sinagra G, De Caterina R. Additional value of T1 and T2 mapping techniques for early detection of myocardial involvement in scleroderma. Int J Cardiol. 2023 Apr 1;376:139–46.

70. Panopoulos S, Mavrogeni S, Vlachopoulos C, et al. Cardiac magnetic resonance imaging before and after therapeutic interventions for systemic sclerosis-associated myocarditis. Rheumatology (Oxford). 2023;62(4):1535–42.

10

Idiopathic inflammatory myositis

KATHLEENA D'ANNA AND CHRISTINA DOWNEY

INTRODUCTION

There are several different types of immune inflammatory myositis (IIM), each of which has a distinct clinical and pathological characteristic which defines them as distinctive entities. The most common and well-characterized are dermatomyositis (DM) and polymyositis (PM). Many other diseases may be mistaken for inflammatory myopathy, including but not limited to muscular dystrophy, metabolic mimickers, infections including bacterial and viral, hypothyroidism, vitamin D deficiency, diabetes, and drug or toxin-induced myopathies. Diagnosis should be guided by a detailed history and physical exam paired with antibody testing, imaging, and in some cases muscle biopsy. Patients with suspected IIM should also undergo comprehensive screening for associated autoimmune conditions and malignancies. Inflammatory myopathies at times co-exist with other connective tissue diseases such as mixed connective tissue disease, polyarteritis nodosa, sarcoidosis, scleroderma, systemic lupus erythematosus, rheumatoid arthritis, and Sjögren's disease.[1,2]

The pathogenicity of DM is not completely understood, but a major theory describes the directed effect of inflammatory cell infiltration into the muscle tissue. This immune complex binding to endothelium cells leads to downstream activation of the complement system and cell lysis mediated by membrane attack complex resulting in necrosis. Histological evaluation of patients with myositis has identified a predominance of CD4+ and CD8+ T cells, B cells, macrophages, and dendritic cells. These proinflammatory cells lead to the expression of additional cytokines such as IFN-y, IL-1b, TNF-a, and TGF-b, as well as chemokines contribute to an indirect effect of continued inflammation affecting the microvasculature.[3] Thickening of endothelial cells capillaries and venules due to the abundance of inflammatory cells, cytokines, and chemokines increases adhesion molecules and decreases capillaries in muscle tissue leading to the typical histologic finding of perivascular atrophy found in DM.

Some newer theories are targeting IFN as the main contributor of inflammatory damage. While DM is thought to be complement mediated, PM and inclusion body myositis (IBM) have been found to be T-cell-mediated processes. Histological biopsies frequently show muscle infiltration with CD8+ and CD4+ T-cells in the muscle tissues. The cytotoxic T-cell targets MHC class I antigen-expressing muscle fibers, and this interaction allows the T-Cell MHC-1 complex to act as an antigen-presenting cell (APC), prompting further cytotoxic T-cell activation, which then leads to fiber necrosis.[3,4] Genetic risk factors have also been identified, with different ethnic groups associating with different haplotypes, showcasing the complexity of the pathogenesis of the diseases.[5] Some known risk factors for the disease are viruses, bacteria, parasites, drugs, UV radiation, smoking, and malignancies.

DOI: 10.1201/9781003386711-10

Dermatomyositis (DM)

DM typically presents with symmetric proximal muscle weakness typically developing over weeks to months with two peaks of onset: 14 years and 45 years. Women are twice as likely to be affected as men. In adult-onset DM, between 15 and 27% of patients will receive a malignancy diagnosis within five years of diagnosis. NXP2 and anti-p-155/TIF1-γ autoantibodies have a higher association with malignancy. Skin disease is prevalent in patients with anti-SAE antibody positivity.[6] On biopsy inflammatory, infiltrates occur predominantly at perivascular sites or within the interfascicular septae of the muscle fibers, with B cells and CD4 cells predominating. One of the hallmark features of DM is a distribution of atrophic, degenerating, and

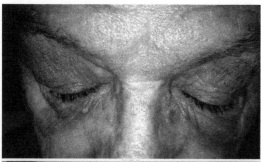
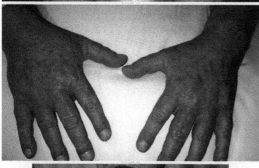
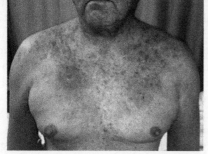

Figure 10.1 Skin manifestations of dermatomyositis. (© ACR 2020.)[9]

regenerating fibers at the periphery of the fascicle.[7] Anti-Mi2 antibody-positive DM patients have particularly pronounced muscle damage with more necrosis found on muscle biopsy.[8]

Skin lesions are a hallmark feature of DM (see Figure 10.1). Common skin manifestations include the following: Heliotropic rash, which is a rash involving the periorbital region with a dusky blue/purple discoloration, edema of the eyelids, Gottron's papules over extensor surfaces, subcutaneous calcifications, hyperpigmentation of the extensor surfaces of joints such as elbows and knees, photosensitive rashes, and others.

Other manifestations include arthritis, Raynaud's phenomenon, dysphagia, and interstitial lung diseases. While rashes may appear red or pink on lighter colored skin, it is important to recognize that DM rashes look different in patients of color. The rashes of DM in darker skin tones are more violaceous and hyperpigmented which may be associated with loss of pigmentation in some areas (Figure 10.2).[10]

Some patients with DM may have a subset known as amyopathic DM, where muscle weakness is not found. However, extra-cutaneous manifestations such as interstitial lung disease (ILD) and cardiovascular disease (CVD) may still be present. Clinically amyopathic disease can be associated with anti-MDA5 antibodies, which can herald rapidly progressing ILD in this phenotype.[11]

Polymyositis (PM)

Like DM, PM presents with symmetric proximal muscle weakness that develops over weeks to months but can present acutely. Weakness is most notable in the pelvic girdle, proximal shoulders, and neck flexors; however, lack of rashes is a distinguishing feature.[12] Creatinine kinase values may be increased up to 50 fold, while the disease is active and inflammatory markers, liver enzymes, and ANA levels may also be markedly elevated on presentation.[13] On muscle biopsy, mononuclear inflammatory cells, predominantly cytotoxic CD8+ T cells, are typically found as cellular infiltrations occurring at the perimysium.[7] Myocardial biopsy in a patient with PM is noted in Figure 10.3. PM is more common in Black populations than in White populations and the age of onset is typically between 50 and 60 years.[14] Like DM, PM is twice as common in women as in men.

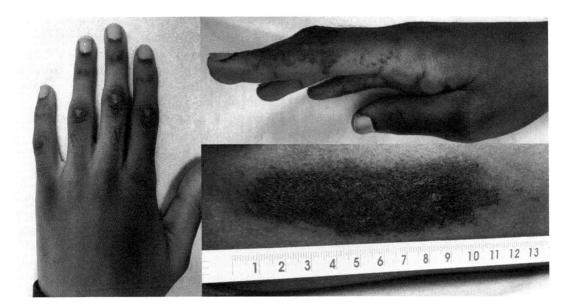

Figure 10.2 Skin manifestations of dermatomyositis in darker skin tone. (© ACR 2020)[9]

Immune-mediated necrotizing myopathy (IMNM)

This distinct disease process is characterized by severe proximal muscle weakness, high creatinine kinase levels, rarity of systemic symptoms or other systemic organ involvement, and relatively favorable response to treatment.[15] Immune-mediated necrotizing myopathy (IMNM) is composed of antibody-negative, anti-SRP positive, and anti-HMGCR positive subsets. Anti-HMGCR antibodies may occur in the absence of exposure to statin

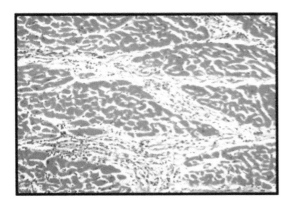

Figure 10.3 Cellular infiltrate composed predominantly of lymphocytes found in the myocardial septa. The myocardial fibers themselves appear normal, and no evidence of degeneration is seen. (© ACR 2020.)[29]

medications. Antibody-negative IMNM patients may be at higher risk of coexistent malignancy.[16] Muscle histology is characterized by randomly distributed necrotic muscle fibers along with fibers in various stages of regeneration, absence, or very few mononuclear cells.[7] The age distribution of disease onset is typically between 50 and 60 years with a slight female predominance. Younger patients tend to have more pronounced disease. The incidence is thought to be about 1–100,000 people.[17]

Anti-synthetase syndrome

Myositis, ILD, calcinosis, inflammatory arthritis, Raynaud's and mechanic's hands are hallmarks of anti-synthetase syndrome.[18] There are a host of autoantibodies associated with this syndrome, aminoacyl-transfer RNA synthetase (Jo-1) being the most common. Anti-PL-7, anti-PL-12, anti-OJ, anti-EJ, anti-KS, anti-Wa, anti-YRS, and anti-Zo are all associated with this distinct clinical entity.[4] Patients with an atypical Rheumatoid Arthritis picture and ILD should be screened for anti-synthetase syndrome as 5–8% of patients will manifest as an overlap syndrome.[19] The age of onset is between 50 and 60 years. The incidence is estimated to be around 0.56 per 100,000, prevalence 9 per 100,000. Male and female distribution is almost equal, although some studies have shown female predominance.[20]

Inclusion body myositis (IBM)

In contrast to the other IIM, IBM is distinguished by asymmetric muscle weakness typically affecting the hand flexors and knee extensors and insidious onset of disease; this form of IIM is exclusively diagnosed in those over the age of 50 years and has a gender distribution skewing heavily male.[21] This form of IIM does not respond well to treatment and many patients may develop significant dysphagia requiring G-tube placement and parenteral nutrition.[21] As such, patients with IBM suffer a higher rate of mortality than those with other forms of IIM. IBM is not associated with underlying malignancy; however, several studies have shown an association with other autoimmune diseases specifically rheumatoid arthritis and Sjögren's disease.[21]

The pathologic hallmark of IBM muscle biopsy includes intracellular amyloid deposits, abnormal protein aggregates, and rimmed vacuoles identified with fluorescence-enhanced Congo red staining.[7,21] IBM is a rare form of myositis, with prevalence estimated to be between 0.1 and 13 per 100,000 people.[21] Difficulties in establishing a diagnosis are attributed to the broad range of the prevalence. New advances in diagnostic modalities are helping to identify more cases so more recent studies show an increase in prevalence than prior. The discovery of the 5NT1A antibody, which is 95% sensitive, has aided with diagnosis of this disease.[22]

Cardiac involvement in myositis

Overtly, the cardiovascular system is clinically affected in patients with IIM in approximately 9% of cases; connective tissue disease overlap syndromes are more likely to involve the heart, and IBM is the least likely.[23] Subclinical involvement has been reported to be as high as 72% of IIM cases.[24]

Common cardiac manifestations in the IIMs are CVD and accelerated atherosclerosis.[25] Diabetes and hypertension occur at higher rates in patients with IIM than in the general population; 29 and 62% vs. 4 and 9.4%, respectively. Treatment with corticosteroids plays a role in the development of these comorbidities. This translates to an increased risk of mortality, on the order of 75%.[26]

One-fifth of DM hospitalizations in the United States are attributable to atherosclerotic CVD. While hospitalized, these patients are twice as likely to succumb to their disease than those without DM or those with DM without CVD.[27] Congestive heart failure, myocardium pathology, conduction abnormalities, ST-T segment changes, left ventricular diastolic dysfunction, and atrial fibrillation all have been described in IIM.[24] Clinically, some myositis-specific antibodies can portend different cardiac manifestations. Most notably, older studies have identified anti-SRP antibodies as having an increased risk of cardiac involvement; however, more recent studies have refuted this, and the connection is believed to be due to small sample size in previous cohorts.[28] Cardiac complications including heart failure, myocardial infarction, and arrhythmia are among the main contributors of all-cause mortality in patients with IIM. The driving factor in cardiovascular involvement in IIM is likely multifactorial. Some studies have linked the underlying systemic inflammation with local inflammation affecting the myocardium leading to increased risk and susceptibility to traditional risk factors such as DM, HTN, and HLD. Most of the available data on cardiac manifestations in IIM comes from patients with DM and PM.

Pericarditis

Pericarditis and pericardial effusion have been found to be present in 12.3 to 17% of cases. Effusions are typically small to moderate and are associated with comorbid pulmonary fibrosis, presence of JO-1 antibody, the anti-synthetase syndrome, and anti-Ro-52 antibody presence.[30,31] Pericarditis in IIM tends to be asymptomatic, which likely contributes to the low number of identified cases.[32] Clinically, pericarditis in myositis patients presents as in non-myositis patients with chest tightness.

Myocarditis

The myocardium is the most frequently involved cardiac structure in IIM, found in about 25–30% of patients in postmortem studies.[33] Similar perivascular inflammation as seen in skeletal muscles leads to fibrosis and small vessel disease of the myocardium. Mononuclear cells in the endomysium and perivascular infiltrates are seen on autopsy specimens.[34] Medial smooth muscle hyperplasia with little to no intimal proliferation may also contribute to left ventricular dysfunction.

Diagnosis can be made with cardiac MRI. At least two of three cardiac MRI abnormalities are required to diagnose myocarditis: myocardial edema on T2-weighted sequences, capillary leak, and fibrosis (as assessed on gadolinium enhancement sequences).[35]

Cardiomyopathy

The heart chamber most likely to be affected by cardiomyopathy in IIM is the left ventricle (LV). In some cohorts, LV dysfunction is present in up to 76.5% of patients and right ventricle involvement is present in 58.5% of cases.[35,36] Disease duration is positively correlated with the development of cardiomyopathy, as is the presence of antimitochondrial, anti-MDA5, and anti-Ro antibodies.[37,38] These result from direct pathogenesis of the inflammatory process leading to degeneration of myocytes and subsequent tissue fibrosis.[39] This fibrosis is also partially responsible for the conduction abnormalities described below. Some studies have found diastolic heart failure to be a long-term consequence of IIM and rarely the degree of dilation may warrant the need for a heart transplant.[39]

Conduction abnormalities

Inflammatory infiltration of cardiac muscle and subsequent fibrotic tissue formation leads to a variety of conduction abnormalities, such as first-degree atrioventricular block, second- and third-degree heart block, prolonged PR-intervals, ventricular premature beats, low-voltage QRS complexes, left atrial enlargement, and right bundle branch block.[32] Histopathological changes similar to those in the myocardium were also observed in the conducting system, including lymphocytic infiltration, fibrosis of the sinoatrial node, and contraction band necrosis at autopsy of myositis patients.[34]

On ECG, this can present as non-specific ST-T or T-wave changes but can also manifest as sinus brady or tachycardia. Rarely patients may require a pacemaker due to this involvement. Other arrhythmias seen in patients with IIM are atrial fibrillation, ectopic atrial rhythm, sinus arrhythmia, supraventricular tachycardia, extrasystoles, premature ventricular complexes, and non-sustained ventricular tachycardia.[24] The chronic inflammation of IIMs and many other rheumatic diseases is linked with accelerated atherosclerosis. This in combination with the risk of cerebrovascular accident (CVA) in patients with atrial fibrillation should alert clinicians to the need for a high clinical suspicion for this conduction disorder. Even in subclinical atrial fibrillation, the risk of CVAs is very high, with a hazard ratio of 2.49; 95% CI, 1.28–4.85; p=0.007.[40]

Because one-fifth of hospitalizations in the United States for patients with DM were associated with an atherosclerosis diagnosis or procedure, and because DM patients are twice as likely to die while hospitalized than those without DM, increased cardiovascular monitoring for arrhythmias while hospitalized may be warranted, though a cost-effectiveness study or outcomes study has not been performed to date.[27]

Valvular disease

Clinically significant valvular insufficiency is rare. Typical involvement includes thickened leaflets, mitral valve prolapse, and mitral and aortic valve stenosis.[34,41]

Pulmonary HTN has been found on ECHO, but the overall incidence is unknown.[33]

Vasculitis

DM is characterized by disease-identifying vascular changes that manifest on the skin. Changes in blood vessels can present as any number of skin findings – including but not limited to Gottron's sign, Gottron's papules, V sign, Shawl sign, and heliotrope rash. Autopsy evaluation of blood vessels shows vessel wall enlargement.[34] It is likely that these vascular changes contribute significantly to progressive CVD.

Cardiovascular disease (CVD) and accelerated atherosclerosis

There is a well-known increased risk of CVD in chronic inflammatory rheumatic diseases such as systemic lupus erythematosus and rheumatoid arthritis.[42] The working hypothesis for accelerated atherosclerosis in IIM is associated with the chronic inflammatory state[42] and consequential endothelial dysfunction contributing to the pathogenesis of atherosclerosis.[43] Chronic activation of the inflammatory response can generate damaging free radicals which cause vascular damage, impair the body's innate anticoagulation pathway, and inhibit fibrinolytic processes contributing to a prothrombotic state. This association in IIM has been gaining momentum in recent years. A large meta-analysis published in 2021 found that IIM patients have an increased risk of CVD when compared with the general population (RR = 2.19, 95% CI: 1.40–3.42).[44] Another found a similar result; patients with IIM had a 2.24-fold increased risk of CAD.[43] The studies examined also found a higher prevalence of traditional CVD risk factors in patients with IIM with hypertension carrying an odds ratio of 1.44, diabetes mellitus 1.67, and dyslipidemia 1.48.[44] Other investigations have corroborated this coexistence of cardiovascular risk factors in patients with IIM.[35,45]

Reluctance for patients with IIM to take cholesterol-lowering medications for their potential to cause myalgia and trigger myositis may be part of this association. Still, the role of exercise cannot be overlooked. It has been established that aerobic exercise is an effective addition to pharmaceutical treatment for hypertension, diabetes mellitus, and dyslipidemia.[46–48] Patients with IIM are typically sidelined from the ability to aerobically exercise due to a variety of factors. Weakness in the proximal muscles, disease-related fatigue, reduced cardiovascular capacity due to interstitial lung disease and fibrosis, arthritis, the need to avoid direct sun exposure as a trigger for rashes, and conduction abnormalities have all been cited as barriers to exercise prescriptions in this group of patients.[49]

In addition to myocardial infarctions, IIM patients are also at an elevated risk for cerebrovascular events, as high as a 1.61-fold increased risk beyond that of the general population.[43] As described above, this is particularly relevant in a population at increased risk for atrial fibrillation and other conduction abnormalities. Ischemic strokes and thromboembolic strokes have both been tied to IIM, with DM being a particular risk factor for ischemic CVA.[50] A meta-analysis found that the risk of ischemic stroke is increased by 49% over the standard risk in Asian patients,[50] illustrating the need to aggressively control risk factors in a team-based approach when caring for IIM patients.

Part of the challenge of caring for IIM patients is the mainstay treatments such as glucocorticoids which increase the burden of cardiovascular and cerebrovascular disease as corticosteroid use itself confers an increased risk of atherosclerotic disease. Further research is needed to increase the availability of non-glucocorticoid immunosuppressants so the lifetime exposure to glucocorticoids can be reduced in this patient population.

Detection and monitoring

Practice guidelines do not currently support baseline EKG or echocardiograms for patients diagnosed with inflammatory myositis due to the non-specific nature of cardiac involvement and lack of clear sensitivity/specificity of results.[32] Instead, a symptom-based diagnostic approach is used to guide the detection of cardiovascular involvement. The mainstay of treatment for myositis is corticosteroids and immunosuppression medications, the former of which can increase the risk of cardiac-associated risk factors. Recent advances in imaging technology, such as the availability of cardiac MRI and myocardial and skeletal mapping, are helping to reach diagnostic conclusions as well as aid more accurately in distinguishing between acute viral myocarditis and IIM induced.[51]

A particular challenge has arisen in the years after the discovery of the SARS-CoV-2 virus (COVID) and subsequent pandemic. The acute myocarditis of COVID can be nearly indistinguishable from that of IIM and COVID has been suggested as a trigger for IIM, making the sequence of diagnosis nearly impossible.[52] Access to non-invasive techniques is especially useful in the post-COVID pandemic era where overlap and increased frequency of viral myocarditis add an additional challenge to the accuracy of the diagnosis of true IIM.

Echocardiogram screening should be utilized promptly if clinical cardiac symptoms are present in a patient with IIM to evaluate for potential structural abnormalities. The use of Cardiac MRI with Gadolinium is being used to detect early myocarditis[33] in newly diagnosed IIM patients with cardiac symptoms to help guide therapy for these patients.[53] While echocardiograms are more convenient and less expensive, cardiac MRI is more precise at determining if there is active myocardial involvement than echocardiogram or cardiac muscle scintigraphy.[24]

Treatments and interventions

Treatment is tailored to the type of myositis; most are managed with a combination of immunosuppression medications. Typically, the mainstay of treatment is glucocorticoids with the addition of a steroid-sparing agent. Agents include methotrexate, azathioprine, mycophenolate, IVIG, and rituximab.[54] There are varying levels of evidence suggesting that cardiac manifestations of IIM are improved with treatment of the underlying myositis; however, there is also ample evidence to suggest the contrary. One promising case report showed a reversal of multifocal atrial tachycardia, premature ventricular excitations, and Mobitz block after therapy with glucocorticoids and rituximab.[55] Other studies have shown an improvement in the ejection fraction and myocardial enhancement on cardiac MRI after treatment with glucocorticoids and immunosuppressant therapy.[56]

It cannot be overlooked that the mainstay of therapy for IIMs, corticosteroids, also increases the risk of comorbidities associated with CVD and is a risk factor in and of itself, with an adjusted risk ratio of 1.5 for new-onset arterial thromboembolic events in persons with inflammatory myopathy.[57] However, treatment with disease-modifying antirheumatic drugs (DMARDs) reduces the risk of CVD by about half.[58] This points to the need for prompt recognition of IIM disease and speedy initiation of DMARD and/or biologic therapy in these patients.

Members of Black, Indigenous, and People of Color communities are often under-represented in textbooks, with a 2020 review finding only 4–18% of pathology images representing darker skin tones.[59] Delay in IIM diagnosis coupled with an increased risk for poorer CVD outcomes in non-Hispanic Black people, even when controlling for socioeconomic status, makes the need for increased awareness of these diseases and their ill effects on the cardiovascular system urgent.[60]

To improve cardiovascular outcomes in patients who may be severely limited by their ability to conduct aerobic exercise and who are sabotaged by the treatment crucial for controlling acute disease symptoms, IIM patients must modify their CVD risk through other lifestyle interventions. Adhering to a healthful dietary pattern has been found to be independently protective against CVD, with the best evidence for the Alternative Healthy Eating Index and the Healthy Eating Index 2015.[61]

Gastrointestinal involvement of IIM such as dysphagia may interfere with some dietary interventions. Sleep disturbance is another significant risk factor for myocardial infarction, CVAs, hypertension, and a host of other risk factors.[62] Night pain may be preventing patients with IIM from getting adequate quality sleep and this should be screened for.

Psychological health has been gaining increasing attention as a significant effector of CVD risk, including a negative correlation with depression and loneliness.[63] There has long been a known association between rheumatic diseases and the development of depression, including IIMs. IIM tends to strike people when they are still of working age and can impact their quality of life drastically.[64] Inability to participate in social events, change in appearance, side effects of therapy, pain, and disability all contribute to the development of depression and in some cases isolation. Loneliness is an independent risk factor for an increased risk of CVD, CVA, and all-cause mortality.[29] Screening for depression and social isolation is critical to reducing the risk of CVD in not just patients with IIM, but all patients.

CONCLUSION

Idiopathic inflammatory myopathy is a complex and multifaceted group of disease processes focusing on but not limited to subacute muscle weakness and muscle inflammatory pathology. However, as is the case with most rheumatic disease, nearly every organ system may be affected including the cardiovascular system. Clinicians must have knowledge of possible phenotypes of this disease and be vigilant for the development of Interstitial lung disease, cutaneous manifestations including vasculitis, dysphagia and other gastrointestinal pathology, and cardiovascular involvement.

Patients face difficulties in many aspects of the disease process including accurate and prompt diagnosis. Recent innovations and advancements of biomarkers and imaging modalities are working to narrow this gap. Chronic inflammation along with systemic toxicity associated with mainstay treatment of most IIM drives up an already heightened prevalence of accelerated atherosclerosis and subsequent CVD. New insight and appreciation on the benefit of modifiable risk factors of CVD in patients with IIM are needed moving forward to improve the quality and longevity of these patients. Already faced with challenging circumstances from the disease itself as well and the treatments, many patients experience social, mental, and economic limitations in various aspects of their lives. Further research, and education both in the patient and physician community, is a necessity to reduce the burden and disability of patients with IIM.

REFERENCES

1. Amato AA, Barohn RJ. Idiopathic inflammatory myopathies. Neurol Clin. 1997;15:615–648.

2. Foote RA, Kimbrough SM, Stevens J. Lupus myositis. Muscle Nerve. 1982;5:65–68.

3. Krathen MS, Fiorentino D, Werth VP. Dermatomyositis. Curr Dir Autoimmun. 2008;10:313–332. https://doi.org/10.1159/000131751

4. Uruha A, Suzuki S, Nishino I. Diagnosis of dermatomyositis: autoantibody profile and muscle pathology. Clin Exp Neuroimmunol. 2017;8:302–312. https://doi.org/10.1111/cen3.12419

5. Firestein G, Budd R, Gabriel D, McInnes I, O'Dell J. Kelley and Firestein's Textbook of Rheumatology. Tenth Edition. Elsevier; 2017.

6. Albayda J, Mecoli C, Casciola-Rosen L, Danoff SK, Lin CT, Hines D, Gutierrez-Alamillo L, Paik JJ, Tiniakou E, Mammen AL, Christopher-Stine L. A North American cohort of anti-SAE dermatomyositis: clinical phenotype, testing, and review of cases. ACR Open Rheumatol. 2021 May;3(5):287–294.

7. Vattemi G, Mirabella M, Guglielmi V, et al. Muscle biopsy features of idiopathic inflammatory myopathies and differential diagnosis. Auto Immun Highlights. 2014;5(3):77–85. https://doi.org/10.1007/s13317-014-0062-2

8. Fornaro M, Girolamo F, Cavagna L, Franceschini F, Giannini M, Amati A, Lia A, Tampoia M, D'Abbicco D, Maggi L, Fredi M. Severe muscle damage with myofiber necrosis and macrophage infiltrates characterize anti-Mi2 positive dermatomyositis. Rheumatology. 2021;60(6):2916–2926.

9. American College of Rheumatology DAM. Images.rheumatology.org. 2024. images.rheumatology.org/bp/#/assets. Accessed 3 Mar. 2024.

10. Dugan EM, Huber AM, Miller FW, Rider LG, International Myositis Assessment and Clinical Studies Group. Photoessay of the cutaneous manifestations of the idiopathic inflammatory myopathies. Dermatol Online J. 2009;15(2):1.

11. McHugh NJ, Targoff IN. Role of ANA and myositis autoantibodies in diagnosis. In: Managing Myositis: A Practical Guide. Springer; 2020:167–174.

12. Bohan A, Peter JB. Polymyositis and dermatomyositis (first of two parts). N Engl J Med. 1975 Feb 13;292(7):344–347.

13. Milisenda JC, Selva-O'Callaghan A, Grau JM. The diagnosis and classification of polymyositis. J Autoimmun. 2014 Feb 1; 48:118–121.

14. Oddis C, Conte C, Steen V. Incidence of polymyositis-dermatomyositis: a 20 year study of hospital diagnosed cases in Allegheny County, PA 1963–1982. J Rheumatol. 1990;17:1329–1334.

15. Kao AH, Lacomis D, Lucas M, Fertig N, Oddis CV. Anti-signal recognition particle autoantibody in patients with and patients without idiopathic inflammatory myopathy. Arthritis Rheum. 2004;50(1):209–215. https://doi.org/10.1002/art.11484

16. Pinal-Fernandez I, Casal-Dominguez M, Mammen AL. Immune-mediated necrotizing myopathy. Curr Rheumatol Rep. 2018 Mar 26;20(4):21. https://doi.org/10.1007/s11926-018-0732-6

17. Khan NAJ, Khalid S, Ullah S, Malik MU, Makhoul S. Necrotizing autoimmune myopathy: a rare variant of idiopathic inflammatory myopathies. J Investig Med High Impact Case Rep. 2017;5(2): 2324709617709031. https://doi.org/10.1177/2324709617709031

18. Zanframundo G, Faghihi-Kashani S, Scirè CA, Bonella F, Corte TJ, Doyle TJ, Fiorentino D, Gonzalez-Gay MA, Hudson M, Kuwana M, Lundberg IE. Defining anti-synthetase syndrome: a systematic literature review. Clin Exp Rheumatol. 2022 Feb 25;40(2):309–319.

19. Cojocaru M, Cojocaru IM, Chicos B. New insights into antisynthetase syndrome. Maedica (Bucur). 2016;11(2):130–135.

20. Coffey C, Wang L, Duong S, Hulshizer C, Crowson C, Ryu J, Ernste F. Incidence of antisynthetase syndrome and risk of malignancy in a population-based cohort (1998-2019) [abstract]. Arthritis Rheumatol. 2021;73 (suppl 9). https://acrabstracts.org/abstract/incidence-of-antisynthetase-syndrome-and-risk-of-malignancy-in-a-population-based-cohort-1998-2019/. Accessed April 18, 2023.

21. Shelly S, Mielke MM, Mandrekar J, et al. Epidemiology and natural history of inclusion body myositis: a 40-year population-based study. Neurology. 2021;96(21): e2653–e2661. https://doi.org/10.1212/WNL.0000000000012004

22. Maher K. Inflammatory myopathy. In: Neuromuscular Pathology Made Easy. 2021 Mar 18 (pp. 159–180). CRC Press.

23. Lilleker JB, Vencovsky J, Wang G, et al. The EuroMyositis registry: an international collaborative tool to facilitate myositis research. Ann Rheum Dis. 2018;77(1):30–39.

24. Opinc AH, Makowski MA, Łukasik ZM, et al. Cardiovascular complications in patients with idiopathic inflammatory myopathies: does heart matter in idiopathic inflammatory myopathies?. Heart Fail Rev. 2021;26:111–125. https://doi.org/10.1007/s10741-019-09909-8

25. Limaye V, Hakendorf P, Woodman RJ, et al. Mortality and its predominant causes in a large cohort of patients with biopsy-determined inflammatory myositis. Intern Med J. 2012;42(2):191–198.

26. Limaye VS, Lester S, Blumbergs P, et al. Idiopathic inflammatory myositis is associated with a high incidence of hypertension and diabetes mellitus. Int J Rheum Dis. 2010;13(2):132–137.

27. Linos E, Fiorentino D, Lingala B, et al. Atherosclerotic cardiovascular disease and dermatomyositis: an analysis of the nationwide inpatient sample survey. Arthritis Res Ther. 2013;15:R7.

28. Hengstman GJ, Brouwer R, Vree Egberts WTM, et al. Clinical and serological characteristics of 125 Dutch myositis patients. Myositis specific autoantibodies aid in the differential diagnosis of the idiopathic inflammatory myopathies. J Neurol. 2002 Jan;249(1):69–75. https://doi.org/10.1007/pl00007850

29. Hodgson S, Watts I, Fraser S, Roderick P, Dambha-Miller H. Loneliness, social isolation, cardiovascular disease and mortality: a synthesis of the literature and conceptual framework. J R Soc Med. 2020 May;113(5):185–192.

30. Wang Y, Zeng Q, Cai X, Meng Y, Zhang C, Fan J, Aibibula M, Feng N, Luo L, Ma X. Pericardial effusion in idiopathic inflammatory myopathies: a cross-sectional study from asia and review of the literature. Int J Immunopathol Pharmacol. 2022 Dec 7;36:03946320221145784.

31. Meudec L, Jelin G, Forien M, Palazzo E, Dieudé P, Ottaviani S. Antisynthetase syndrome and cardiac involvement: a rare association. Joint Bone Spine. 2019;86 (Issue 4):517–518. https://doi.org/10.1016/j.jbspin.2018.09.019

32. Lundberg IE. The heart in dermatomyositis and polymyositis. Rheumatology. October 2006;45, (suppl_4):iv18–iv21. https://doi.org/10.1093/rheumatology/kel311

33. Lu Z, Guo-chun W, Li M, Ning Z. Cardiac involvement in adult polymyositis or dermatomyositis: a systematic review. Clin Cardiol. 2012;35:685–691. https://doi.org/10.1002/clc.22026

34. Denbow CE, Lie JT, Tancredi RG, Bunch TW. Cardiac involvement in polymyositis. Arthritis Rheumatol. 1979;22:1088–1092. https://doi.org/10.1002/art.1780221007

35. Diederichsen LP, Diederichsen AC, Simonsen JA, et al. Traditional cardiovascular risk factors and coronary artery calcification in adults with polymyositis and dermatomyositis: a Danish multicenter study. Arthritis Care Res (Hoboken). 2015;67(6):848–854. https://doi.org/10.1002/acr.22520

36. Rosenbohm A, Buckert D, Gerischer N, Walcher T, Kassubek J, Rottbauer W, Ludolph AC, Bernhardt P. Early diagnosis of cardiac involvement in idiopathic inflammatory myopathy by cardiac magnetic resonance tomography. J Neurol. 2015;262(4):949–956.

37. Matsuo T, Sasai T, Nakashima R, et al. ECG changes through immunosuppressive therapy indicate cardiac abnormality in anti-MDA5 antibody-positive clinically amyopathic dermatomyositis. Front Immunol. 2022;12:765140. https://doi.org/10.3389/fimmu.2021.765140

38. Behan WM, Behan PO, Gairns J. Cardiac damage in polymyositis associated with antibodies to tissue ribonucleoproteins. Br Heart J. 1987;57(2):176–180. https://doi.org/10.1136/hrt.57.2.176

39. Schwartz T, Diederichsen LP, Lundberg IE, et al. Cardiac involvement in adult and juvenile idiopathic inflammatory myopathies. RMD Open. 2016;2:e000291. https://doi.org/10.1136/rmdopen-2016-000291

40. Healey JS, Connolly SJ, Gold MR, Israel CW, Van Gelder IC, Capucci A, Lau CP, Fain E, Yang S, Bailleul C, Morillo CA. Subclinical atrial fibrillation and the risk of stroke. N Engl J Medicine. 2012;366(2):120–129.

41. Badui E, Mintz G, Robles E. El corazón en la dermatomiositis y polimiositis [the heart in dermatomyositis and polymyositis]. Arch Inst Cardiol Mex. 1986;56(1):71–76.

42. Zeller CB, Appenzeller S. Cardiovascular disease in systemic lupus erythematosus: the role of traditional and lupus related risk factors. Curr Cardiol Rev. 2008;4(2):116–122. https://doi.org/10.2174/157340308784245775

43. Ungprasert P, Suksaranjit P, Spanuchart I, Leeaphorn N, Permpalung N. Risk of coronary artery disease in patients with idiopathic inflammatory myopathies: a systematic review and meta-analysis of observational studies. Semin Arthritis Rheum. 2014 Aug;44(1):63–67. https://doi.org/10.1016/j.semarthrit.2014.03.004

44. Qin L, Li F, Luo Q, Chen L, Yang X, Wang H. Coronary heart disease and cardiovascular risk factors in patients with idiopathic inflammatory myopathies: a systemic review and meta-analysis. Front Med (Lausanne). 2022 Jan 14;8:808915. https://doi.org/10.3389/fmed.2021.808915

45. Mizus MC, Tiniakou E. Lipid-lowering therapies in myositis. Curr Rheumatol Rep. 2020 Aug 26;22(10):70. https://doi.org/10.1007/s11926-020-00942-3

46. Saco-Ledo G, Valenzuela PL, Ruiz-Hurtado G, Ruilope LM, Lucia A. Exercise reduces ambulatory blood pressure in patients with hypertension: a systematic review and meta-analysis of randomized controlled trials. J Am Heart Assoc. 2020 Dec 15;9(24):e018487.

47. Kumar AS, Maiya AG, Shastry BA, Vaishali K, Ravishankar N, Hazari A, Gundmi S, Jadhav R. Exercise and insulin resistance in type 2 diabetes mellitus: a systematic review and meta-analysis. Ann Phys Rehabil Med. 2019 Mar 1;62(2):98–103.

48. Zhao S, Zhong J, Sun C, Zhang J. Effects of aerobic exercise on TC, HDL-c, LDL-c and TG in patients with hyperlipidemia: a protocol of systematic review and meta-analysis. Medicine. 2021 Mar 3;100(10):e25103.

49. Andreasson KM. Exercise training in myositis recovery: practical issues and challenges. Indian J Rheumatol. 2023 Mar;4:10–4103.

50. Zhen C, Wang Y, Wang H, Wang X. The risk of ischemic stroke in patients with idiopathic inflammatory myopathies: a systematic review and meta-analysis. Clin Rheumatol. 2021 Oct;40(10):4101–4108.

51. Huber AT, Bravetti M, Lamy J, et al. Non-invasive differentiation of idiopathic inflammatory myopathy with cardiac involvement from acute viral myocarditis using cardiovascular magnetic resonance imaging T1 and T2 mapping. J Cardiovasc Magn Reason. 2018;20:11. https://doi.org/10.1186/s12968-018-0430-6

52. Freund O, Eviatar T, Bornstein G. Concurrent myopathy and inflammatory cardiac disease in COVID-19 patients: a case series and literature review. Rheumatol Int. 2022 May;42(5):905–912.

53. Cheston HJ, Akhoon C, Dutta Roy S, et al. Managing myocarditis in a patient with newly diagnosed dermatomyositis. BMJ Case Rep CP. 2022;15:e246989.

54. Barsotti S, Lundberg IE. Current treatment for myositis. Curr Treatm Opt Rheumatol. 2018;4(4):299–315. https://doi.org/10.1007/s40674-018-0106-2

55. Touma Z, Arayssi T, Kibbi L, Masri AF. Successful treatment of cardiac involvement in dermatomyositis with rituximab. Joint Bone Spine. 2008;75(Issue 3):334–337.

56. Allanore Y, Vignaux O, Arnaud L, Puéchal X, Pavy S, Duboc D, Legmann P, Kahan A. Effects of corticosteroids and immuno-suppressors on idiopathic inflammatory myopathy related myocarditis evaluated by magnetic resonance imaging. Ann Rheum Dis. 2006;65(2):249–252.

57. Tisseverasinghe A, Bernatsky S, Pineau CA. Arterial events in persons with derma-tomyositis and polymyositis. J Rheumatol. 2009;36(9):1943–1946.

58. Roifman I, Beck PL, Anderson TJ, et al. Chronic inflammatory diseases and cardio-vascular risk: a systematic review. Can J Cardiol. 2011;27:174–182.

59. Adelekun A, Onyekaba G, Lipoff JB. Skin color in dermatology textbooks: an updated evaluation and analysis. J Am Acad Dermatol. 2021 Jan 1;84(1):194–196.

60. Karlamangla AS, Merkin SS, Crimmins EM, Seeman TE. Socioeconomic and ethnic dis-parities in cardiovascular risk in the United States, 2001–2006. Ann Epidemiol. 2010 Aug 1;20(8):617–628.

61. Shan Z, Li Y, Baden MY, Bhupathiraju SN, Wang DD, Sun QI, Rexrode KM, Rimm EB, Qi LU, Willett WC, Manson JE. Association between healthy eating patterns and risk of cardiovascular disease. JAMA Intern Med. 2020 Aug 1;180(8):1090–100.

62. Grandner MA, Jackson NJ, Pak VM, Gehrman PR. Sleep disturbance is associated with cardiovascular and metabolic disorders. J Sleep Res. 2012 Aug;21(4):427–433.

63. Levine GN, Cohen BE, Commodore-Mensah Y, Fleury J, Huffman JC, Khalid U, Labarthe DR, Lavretsky H, Michos ED, Spatz ES, Kubzansky LD. Psychological health, well-being, and the mind-heart-body con-nection: a scientific statement from the American Heart Association. Circulation. 2021 Mar 9;143(10):e763–e783.

64. Leclair V, Regardt M, Wojcik S, Hudson M, Canadian Inflammatory Myopathy Study (CIMS). Health-related quality of life (HRQoL) in idiopathic inflammatory myopa-thy: a systematic review. PLoS One. 2016 Aug 9;11(8):e0160753.

11

Vasculitis

BRIAN D. JAROS, ARTEM MINALYAN, AND ANISHA B. DUA

GIANT CELL ARTERITIS

Background/Epidemiology

Giant cell arteritis (GCA) is the most common primary vasculitis worldwide with the incidence varying between 0.3 and 44 cases per 100,000 persons over the age of 50 years (1). Incidence peaks between the ages of 70 and 79 with a female predominance. GCA is characterized by granulomatous arteritis of the temporal artery (2). Involvement of the aorta and its large branches can also be observed. Early pathogenesis involves the activation of vascular dendritic cells that upregulates the activity of CD4+ T cells. The latter differentiate into Th1 and Th17 cells. IL-6 amplifies the differentiation of Th17 cells, resulting in the production of IL-17. Importantly, this pathway is predominant in early GCA and responsive to glucocorticoid (GC) therapy (3). IL-12 and IL-18 are involved in the differentiation of Th1 cells, leading to the release of IFN-γ, which is associated with chronic disease and resistance to GC therapy (4).

Clinical presentation and diagnosis

GCA is subdivided into three groups based on the primary site of the arterial inflammation: cranial GCA (C-GCA), large-vessel (LV)-GCA, and LV-GCA with cranial involvement (5). The majority of patients with C-GCA have unilateral temporal headache. Other symptoms include jaw claudication and visual changes (amaurosis fugax, double vision, blindness). The most specific ocular manifestation is anterior ischemic optic neuropathy. Tenderness with erythema and decreased pulsation over the temporal artery can be present. In LV-GCA, symptoms may include limb claudication, chest or abdominal pain, and constitutional symptoms. Notably, between 40 and 60% of patients with GCA have signs and symptoms of polymyalgia rheumatica (PMR) (6). The ACR/ EULAR 2022 classification criteria use a combination of clinical, laboratory (ESR ≥ 50 mm/h or CRP ≥ 10 mg/L), imaging (color Doppler ultrasound [CDUS], FDG-PET), and biopsy criteria to classify the disease (7).

Cardiac involvement

Cardiac involvement is present in approximately 5% of patients with GCA (8). Several mechanisms have been proposed to explain cardiac ischemic events: (1) vascular inflammation leading to narrowing of the vascular lumen and downstream tissue ischemia; (2) accelerated atherosclerosis due to underlying endothelial dysfunction in the setting of vascular wall inflammation; (3) the impact of GC use (9). Patients with GCA have a higher prevalence of pericarditis when compared to age- and sex-matched controls (1.22 vs 0.33%, respectively) (8). The association is particularly strong among younger patients (age < 70 years). The timing of pericarditis in relation to other findings of GCA is highly variable. The most common pericardial involvement in GCA is pericardial effusion (10).

DOI: 10.1201/9781003386711-11

Despite potential pathophysiologic risk factors, there appears to be no overall increased risk of acute coronary syndrome in patients with GCA compared to controls (11). Greigert et al. reported 13 cases of MI among 251 biopsy-proven GCA patients (12). Surprisingly, only one patient had coronary artery changes suggestive of coronary vasculitis. Patients with LV-GCA are at risk of developing aortic dilation, due to vascular wall weakening secondary to inflammation. Nuenninghoff et al. reported that 18% of patients with GCA developed aortic dilations and/or dissections, most commonly of the thoracic aorta (13). Aortic regurgitation has been reported in patients with ascending aortitis who have subsequent aortic root dilation or aneurysm (14–16). Underlying coronary disease may further increase the risk of aortic dilation (15). The frequency of specific cardiac manifestations in GCA and the other vasculitides discussed in this chapter are presented in Table 11.1.

Treatment

High-dose oral GCs are recommended in GCA patients without cranial ischemia and intravenous (IV) pulse GC if cranial ischemic manifestations are present (amaurosis fugax, vision loss, and stroke) (17). Tocilizumab, an IL-6 inhibitor, use is recommended, concurrently with GC, as part of induction due to its significant steroid-sparing effect (18). In patients with flow-limiting involvement of the vertebral and carotid arteries, the addition of aspirin is a consideration. Revascularization interventions should be a collaborative decision between rheumatology and vascular surgery teams, as well as cardiology, neurology, and interventional radiology, depending on the clinical context.

Table 11.1 Reported cardiac manifestations of vasculitides

Vasculitis	Myocarditis	Pericarditis	Coronary arteritis	Valvular disease	Ascending aortitis	Comments
GCA	✓	✓		✓	✓	~5% cardiac involvement, very rare case reports of coronary arteritis
TAK	✓	✓	✓	✓	✓	Unlike GCA, can cause pulmonary arteritis
KD	✓	✓	✓	✓	✓	Untreated, 25% develop coronary aneurysms
PAN	✓	✓	✓		✓	
EGPA	✓	✓	✓	✓		Cardiomyopathy leading to heart failure in ~18%
GPA/ MPA	✓	✓	✓	✓	✓	Rare involvement overall with more valvular disease reported in GPA > MPA
CV	✓	✓	✓			Rare cardiac involvement
BS	✓	✓	✓	✓	✓	Pulmonary vascular aneurysms can be seen

Key: Green shading indicates typical or well-described involvement. Yellow shading indicates uncommon or less typical but reported involvement. Red shading indicates no described involvement.

Abbreviations: GCA, Giant cell arteritis; TAK, Takayasu arteritis; KD—Kawasaki disease; PAN, Polyarteritis nodosa; EGPA, Eosinophilic granulomatosis with polyangiitis; GPA/MPA, Granulomatosis with polyangiitis/ microscopic polyangiitis; CV, Cryoglobulinemic vasculitis; BS, Behçet syndrome

TAKAYASU ARTERITIS (TAK)

Background/Epidemiology

Takayasu arteritis (TAK) is a large-vessel vasculitis characterized by granulomatous inflammation of the vascular wall. TAK was originally thought to affect predominantly patients of Asian ancestry, but it is now recognized that the incidence varies significantly depending on geographic location. In Japan, the annual incidence of TAK is 1–2 cases per million, whereas in Europe it ranges from 0.4 to 0.8 per million (19–21). Age of onset is usually between 10 and 40 years, with women being more commonly affected.

The pathogenesis of TAK remains poorly understood. Similar to GCA, the pathogenesis of TAK involves the recruitment of CD4+ T cells. However, it has been shown that CD8+ T lymphocytes, NK cells, and B cells also play an important role in the pathogenesis of TAK, unlike in GCA (22). An association with certain HLA alleles has been established, including HLA-B52, which may predict more severe disease in Japanese patients (23). Infectious triggers of TAK have been hypothesized, including potential pathogenic links to HIV and *Mycobacterium tuberculosis* (24,25).

Clinical features and diagnosis

The initial vascular inflammation in TAK is often asymptomatic or manifests with nonspecific systemic symptoms (low-grade fever, weight loss, fatigue). This explains the significant challenge in timely diagnosis of TAK with a reported median delay of 17.5 months (26). This phase is frequently followed by relapsing vascular inflammation that can involve new arterial territories. The chronic ("pulseless") phase is the result of vascular ischemia with corresponding signs and symptoms: limb claudication, cyanosis, lightheadedness, carotidynia, hypertension, weak or absent peripheral pulses, discrepant blood pressure, abdominal pain, and visual changes. Arterial bruits can be auscultated in patients with arterial stenosis, best heard over the subclavian, carotid, and brachial arteries (27). Imaging studies are essential in establishing the diagnosis of TAK. Non-invasive modalities (CT angiography, MR angiography, PET-CT, PET-MR) are preferred. New 2022 ACR/EULAR classification criteria for TAK provide guidance for the research classification of patients, including patient age 60 years or younger (at time of diagnosis) and evidence of vasculitis (the aorta or its branches) with additional clinical and imaging criteria (28). The criteria report that the involvement of multiple, paired arterial territories and the presence of abdominal aortitis involving the renal or mesenteric arteries increase the probability of TAK.

Cardiac involvement

Up to 11% of patients with TAK have coronary artery lesions and, rarely, coronary involvement may be the only site of arteritis in TAK (29). Three types of coronary lesions have been described: (1) stenotic lesions of the ostial segment; (2) diffuse involvement of the coronary artery; (3) aneurysm of coronary artery.

Unlike GCA, TAK can cause pulmonary arteritis. Among those with concurrent TAK and pulmonary arteritis, around 40% of patients develop pulmonary hypertension (30). Similar to GCA, aortic valve involvement occurs as a result of aortic dilation (31). Myocardial involvement often occurs in patients with coronary involvement, valvular pathology, and pulmonary vascular disease in the setting of TAK.

Treatment

In patients with active, severe TAK, initiation of high-dose oral GC is recommended (17). IV pulse GC should be considered in patients with life- or organ-threatening disease. The addition of a steroid-sparing agent (methotrexate [MTX], azathioprine [AZA], or tumor necrosis factor inhibitors [TNFi]) to minimize GC-related toxicity is recommended. In patients with cranial or vertebrobasilar arterial involvement, antiplatelet therapy should be considered. Inflammation of the vessel wall can be asymptomatic, highlighting the importance of regular, non-invasive imaging, though optimal imaging intervals are individualized. New vascular inflammation in clinically asymptomatic patients should be treated with immunosuppressive therapy (32). Surgical treatment is challenging, and, in most cases, medical management is preferred over surgical intervention. Surgical intervention is considered in high-risk (concern for dissection or rupture) aneurysmal dilation, severe aortic regurgitation, or aortic coarctation (33). When feasible, active inflammation should be controlled prior to surgery. Additionally, when planning arterial bypass surgeries, it is important to avoid inflamed vessels when performing repositioning since it can lead to poor vascular flow outcomes. Whenever a surgical approach is pursued, the use of GC in the perioperative period should be considered (34).

KAWASAKI DISEASE (KD)

Background/Epidemiology

Kawasaki disease (KD) is a medium-vessel vasculitis, primarily of childhood. The majority of patients are diagnosed at age 5 or younger, though cases occurring throughout teenage years have been described (35,36). Despite its occurrence in pediatric patients, KD can have implications into adulthood and remains the leading cause of acquired heart disease in children in the developed world (37). The incidence of KD varies geographically, with data from Japan, South Korea, and China indicating overall higher rates of disease compared to those of North America or European countries (38–40). The highest incidence, reported in Japan, is estimated at 1 in 100 children by age 5 (39). This risk seems to be conferred among children with Japanese ancestry living outside of Japan, as demonstrated by epidemiologic studies of KD in the United States (41). The sustained risk, regardless of current location of inhabitance, suggests that genetic background plays some role in the disease. Antecedent viral illness may serve as an environmental risk factor given peak rates of disease during the winter months in the extratropical northern hemisphere; however, no specific pathogen has been identified (42).

Clinical features and diagnosis

The diagnosis of KD is primarily clinical and based on a constellation of major features seen in Figure 11.1. Given the cardiac morbidity and mortality associated with untreated disease, a high index of clinical suspicion is prudent for patients with partial disease features who may not fully meet formal diagnostic criteria (37,43). Labs are nonspecific and show general signs of inflammation, including elevated acute phase reactants, leukocytosis, and thrombocytosis.

Cardiac involvement

Involvement of the coronary arteries is paramount to the morbidity and mortality associated with KD. Dilation of the coronaries occurs in roughly one out of every four to five untreated KD patients (37). Subclinical abnormalities have been described in around 50% of patients (44). Degree of dilation is variable, and even large aneurysms may be asymptomatic until impairments in flow result in thrombosis and/or cardiac ischemia (37). Transthoracic echocardiogram (TTE) remains the gold standard for early, noninvasive detection of potentially silent abnormalities. Aneurysms are typically stratified by size, thus informing the impending risk of clinical consequence. Large or giant aneurysms (≥8 mm) predispose to an increased risk of subsequent events, including acute myocardial infarction, which is the leading cause of death in KD (37). The largest aneurysms are also the least likely to clinically regress. Notably, an initial echocardiogram may be normal if performed within the first week of symptoms. Therefore, surveillance imaging is warranted to reevaluate for the development of vascular inflammation and, even more frequent imaging is needed to monitor the progression of existing lesions. Prompt recognition and treatment of KD aims to reduce the occurrence of acute coronary events in these patients.

Myocardial involvement occurs in over half of patients, often antecedent to coronary artery involvement early in the disease course (45). While acute inflammation may result in ventricular dysfunction, these impairments are typically transient, and long-term functional consequences are unusual (46). Less commonly, myocardial impairment may progress to hemodynamically significant cardiovascular collapse, known as KD shock syndrome. This is typically a warm state with decreased peripheral vascular resistance, different from prototypic cardiogenic shock, and may reflect an overwhelming inflammatory and vasodilatory state. Involvement of the pericardium is described, including the presence of small pericardial effusion, though progression to tamponade is rare (37). The mitral valve is commonly affected with one in four patients demonstrating evidence of mild-moderate mitral regurgitation that is typically transient (47). Severe and long-term valvular damage can result secondary to ischemic injury (48). Aortic root dilation with subsequent aortic regurgitation can occur and may persist over time.

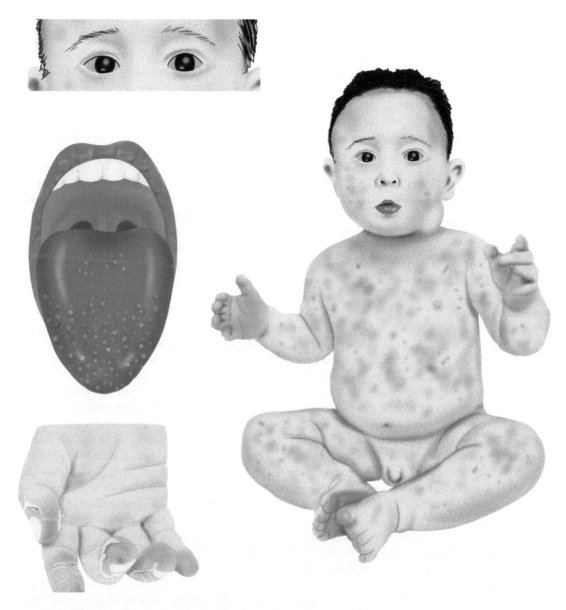

Figure 11.1 Representative illustration of major clinical features of KD, including bilateral conjunctival injection (A), oral erythema and ulceration (B), swelling and erythema of the digits, often with desquamation (C), and erythematous rash of the trunk and extremities (D). Not pictured are cervical lymphadenopathy and self-remitting fever lasting at least five days, which comprise the other major features. (Reprinted with permission from Shutterstock, image 1529252849.)

TTE is an important tool for the evaluation of coronary, valvular, and ventricular abnormalities in KD. In instances of poor TTE visualization or significant cardiac sequelae, advanced imaging, including transesophageal echocardiogram (TEE), computed tomography angiography (CTA), and cardiac magnetic resonance imaging (CMR), as well as conventional angiography, may be considered (37).

Treatment

Time-sensitive initiation of treatment aims to reduce inflammation and prevent long-term consequences of arterial damage. Intravenous immunoglobulin (IVIG) has been shown to reduce the development of coronary artery abnormalities, decreasing mortality by over 95%, and is considered first-line treatment for KD (49–51). A 2 g/kg infusion over 8–12 hours is a typical strategy; however, dosing regimens vary by center. The universal principle is to administer IVIG as soon as the diagnosis is established, given its role in preventing morbidity and mortality. Although ineffective on their own, GCs may be added in patients who are considered to be at risk for resistance to IVIG, given the demonstrated benefit in this select population (52). Persistent fever after 36 hours of IVIG initiation is worrisome for IVIG resistance and warrants the escalation of anti-inflammatory therapy (53). In such patients, the use of infliximab has been successful in case studies and in one randomized trial (54). Additional IVIG doses may also be considered. Further line treatment requires complex multi-disciplinary consideration but may include calcineurin inhibitors, cytotoxic agents, and plasma exchange.

In addition to anti-inflammatory therapy, treatment of KD involves the prevention of thrombosis and the management of cardiac sequelae. Aspirin therapy is recommended during the acute disease period for most patients (37). Depending on the degree and extent of coronary aneurysm, the duration of antiplatelet therapy may be extended and/or escalated to systemic anticoagulation owing to increased thrombotic risk in those with flow-altering vessel wall abnormalities. Development of coronary artery thrombosis may require thrombolysis or mechanical intervention, depending on the degree of occlusion.

Long-term management of KD includes anatomical surveillance, cardiac optimization, and case-based continuation of antiplatelet and/or anticoagulation agents. Even patients whose coronary aneurysms regress in size appear to be at higher long-term cardiovascular risk. This is thought to, at least in part, be related to fibrotic remodeling at aneurysmal sites that affects the elasticity and vascular integrity of the vessel wall (37). Conversely, KD patients who never develop coronary artery aneurysms do not appear to be at increased, long-term cardiovascular risk. Counseling and management of long-term, traditional atherosclerotic risk factors is warranted in all KD patients with cardiac involvement.

POLYARTERITIS NODOSA (PAN)

Background/Epidemiology

Polyarteritis nodosa (PAN) is a necrotizing vasculitis primarily involving medium-sized arteries but sometimes involving small arteries as well. PAN is most common in middle-aged and older adults, though it can affect any age (55). It is a rare disease with an estimated annual incidence rate of 2–9 per million (56).

Clinical features and diagnosis

The diagnosis of PAN relies on a comprehensive history and physical exam due to heterogeneous disease, including cutaneous, renal, neurologic, gastrointestinal, muscular, and cardiovascular manifestations. The lungs are classically spared. Hepatitis B virus is a well-described risk factor, and viral status should be checked. There is currently no recommendation for routine screening for cardiac disease in PAN. CTA and conventional angiography are typically used for the evaluation of the coronary arteries when cardiac disease is suspected. KD must be considered in any child with coronary artery abnormalities undergoing PAN evaluation, as the treatment paradigm for each disease is different (37).

Cardiac involvement

Overt and clinically significant cardiac involvement is rare in PAN. Although uncommon, cardiac involvement portends a worse overall prognosis, similar to many other vasculitides (32). Direct cardiac involvement in PAN most often manifests as coronary arteritis and can result in aneurysmal dilation, thrombotic occlusion, spontaneous dissection, and vasospasm. Cardiac ischemia and infarction with subsequent complications, including ventricular failure, valve rupture, arrhythmia, and shock, are feared complications of these abnormalities. When described in small, postmortem autopsy series, coronary arteritis in PAN patients is reported as high as 50–62% (57,58). This is in contrast to recent clinical data that suggest a more modest occurrence of coronary artery abnormalities, closer to 13% (59). Even lower is the number of PAN patients who experience a myocardial infarction as a result of these abnormalities. This vast discrepancy in incidence may represent the bias of autopsy, which captures a more severe disease phenotype leading to mortality. Since the 1960s, when these autopsy studies were performed, advances in awareness, recognition, and treatment of PAN may have also decreased the number of patients who progress to clinically significant cardiac disease.

Beyond the coronary arteries, involvement of the myocardium and pericardium has been very rarely described in PAN, largely from isolated case reports with biopsy proven vasculitis and immune-mediated invasion of these tissues (58). Remote autopsy series have demonstrated evidence of pericardial disease in almost 25% of PAN patients, which is discordant with the low reported clinical burden of pericarditis in this disease (58). Although immune-mediated cardiomyopathy is uncommon in PAN, heart failure secondary to renal artery involvement with malignant hypertension is well described. Valvulopathy is exceedingly rare.

Treatment

PAN with cardiac manifestations warrants aggressive treatment with a combination of GC and cyclophosphamide (CYC). This approach comes from a number of retrospective studies that observed significantly improved survival outcomes in patients with moderate-severe PAN who were treated with both GC and an additional immunosuppressive agent (commonly CYC) as compared to GC alone (60,61). Patients with end-organ cardiac manifestations should receive pulse dose IV GC followed by a gradual oral taper. Unlike in granulomatosis with polyangiitis (GPA) and microscopic polyangiitis (MPA), rituximab has not demonstrated reliable efficacy in PAN owing to a lack of high-quality evidence.

Cyclophosphamide is the preferred induction agent in patients with severe PAN, including those with cardiac manifestations (62). After induction, transition to another steroid-sparing immunosuppressive agent, such as methotrexate or azathioprine, is generally recommended. Hepatitis B infection, if present, should be treated.

EOSINOPHILIC GRANULOMATOSIS WITH POLYANGIITIS (EGPA)

Background/Epidemiology

EGPA, previously known as Churg–Strauss syndrome, is a necrotizing small-vessel vasculitis characterized by eosinophilic infiltrates and extravascular granulomas. The reported incidence and prevalence of EGPA globally are 1.22 cases per million person-years and 15.27 cases per million individuals (63).

Clinical features and diagnosis

EGPA is classically described in three phases: prodromal, eosinophilic, and vasculitic. Common clinical manifestations include asthma, rhinosinusitis or nasal polyposis, peripheral eosinophilia, and skin or nerve involvement. Cardiac involvement in EGPA is common and may occur early in disease presentation. Approximately 50% of deaths from EGPA are attributed to cardiac etiologies (64).

Cardiac involvement

The frequency of cardiac manifestation ranges widely from 16 to 60%, depending on the EGPA cohort examined and the screening modality performed (64,65). Cardiac involvement appears to be correlated with anti-neutrophil cytoplasm antibody (ANCA)-negativity as well as higher mean eosinophil levels (65). This suggests an ANCA-independent pathophysiologic mechanism driven by eosinophilic-mediated pathways, which may explain the discrepancy of clinical cardiac involvement in EGPA compared to the other ANCA-associated vasculitides.

Cardiac involvement in EGPA is diverse. Cardiomyopathy is the most frequent manifestation, with progression to clinical heart failure in approximately 18% of patients (64,66). Pericarditis with pericardial effusion may occur, including frank tamponade. Valvular involvement has been described (67). In contrast to the medium-vessel vasculitides, frank coronary arterial involvement is uncommon. The cardiac manifestations of EGPA are visually described in Figure 11.2.

Screening studies have demonstrated the presence of cardiac changes in EGPA patients previously thought to be in remission (68). The number

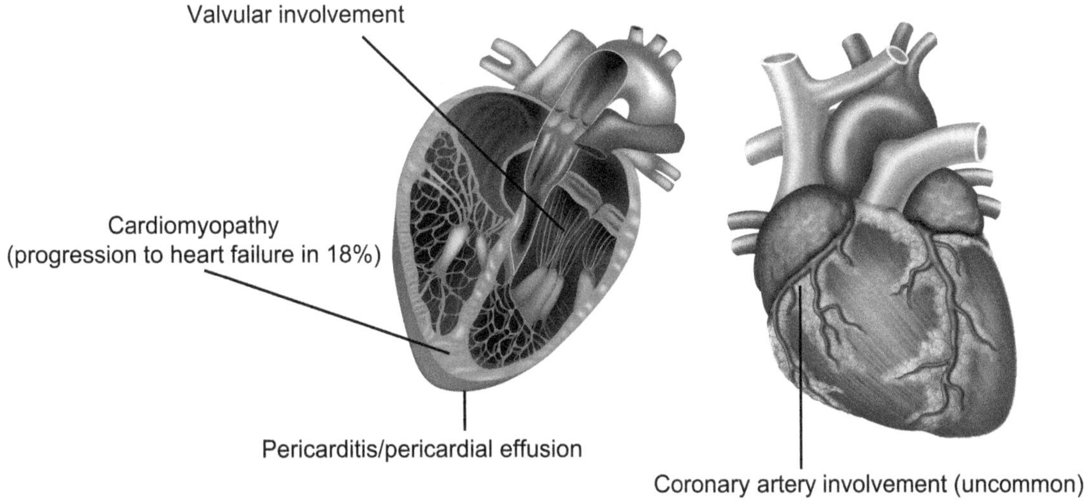

Figure 11.2 Illustration of the potential cardiac involvement in EGPA including disease of the myocardium, pericardium, and valves. Coronary arteritis is uncommon in EGPA. (Reprinted with permission from Shutterstock, images 1110010682 and 1540170977.)

of asymptomatic patients who have been found to have subclinical cardiac involvement ranges from one to two thirds of patients (67). Owing frequency of subclinical involvement, as well as the associated mortality, it is generally agreed that baseline EKG and TTE should be performed in all patients with EGPA. TTE may detect left ventricular systolic or diastolic dysfunction, valvular dysfunction, pericardial effusion or pericarditis, and intracardiac thrombus. CMR is the most sensitive imaging modality for detecting EGPA cardiac involvement, especially when combined with TTE (67). CMR has the advantage of providing a more detailed architectural description as well as differentiating acute, active inflammation from chronic, fibrotic damage. Late gadolinium enhancement (LGE) in the myocardium is characteristic of severe disease. It has been suggested that monitoring interval change in LGE following EGPA treatment may help prognosticate outcomes and guide further intensity of treatment (67). There are ongoing efforts to understand how CMR should be incorporated into the screening of EGPA patients, balancing the study-associated cost with the sensitivity of detection.

Treatment

When the heart is involved in EGPA, disease is considered to be "severe," and aggressive therapy is warranted. Treatment begins with either

IV pulse or high-dose oral GCs, with no data to support one over the other (69). In severe disease, either cyclophosphamide or rituximab is added to GC therapy. The REOVAS study found no difference in remission rates of severe EGPA patients induced with rituximab compared to conventional therapy (70). However, given overall increased experience with cyclophosphamide and because cardiac disease is a significant driver of mortality in EGPA, the ACR/Vasculitis Foundation favors cyclophosphamide induction in EGPA patients with cardiac involvement (69). Mepolizumab, a novel IL-5 targeted antibody, is now approved for use in non-severe and relapsing EGPA. Patients with cardiac disease were not included in the MIRRA trial, which evaluated the efficacy of mepolizumab (71). Thus, at this time, mepolizumab is not recommended for the induction of remission in these patients (69). Following induction of remission in severe disease, maintenance therapy with methotrexate, azathioprine, mepolizumab, or rituximab is recommended (72). Choice of agent is typically based on patient factors, such as organ involvement, comorbidities, and tolerability, given a lack of comparative evidence between these treatments. Optimal treatment duration is unknown, but EGPA patients with prior cardiac involvement should undergo continued surveillance by rheumatology and cardiology providers given the long-term risk of disease relapse.

GRANULOMATOSIS WITH POLYANGIITIS (GPA) AND MICROSCOPIC POLYANGIITIS (MPA)

Background/Epidemiology

GPA and MPA are both necrotizing, small-vessel vasculitides, with GPA showing the histologic presence of granulomatous infiltration. Both diseases are associated with ANCA positivity, and when combined with EGPA, they comprise the ANCA-associated vasculitides. Classically, GPA is associated with cytoplasmic ANCA (c-ANCA) and anti-proteinase 3 (PR3) positivity, while MPA is associated with perinuclear ANCA (p-ANCA) and myeloperoxidase (MPO) positivity. The combined incidence of GPA and MPA appears to be around 3 cases per 100,000 people (73).

Clinical presentation and diagnosis

GPA and MPA often present as pulmonary-renal syndromes. Comparatively, GPA more often affects the upper airway and the ear, nose, and throat. Presentation with constitutional symptoms is common, and nearly any organ system may be affected, including the heart. The estimated prevalence of cardiac involvement in GPA varies vastly depending on the methodology used. The prevalence of clinically apparent cardiac involvement is 3.3–20% (74,75). Other groups have screened for evidence of cardiac involvement using ECG, TTE, cMRI, and PET, regardless of symptoms. Using these methodologies, the estimation of cardiac involvement in GPA can be upward of 61–73%, with a majority of cases being clinically silent (76,77). Cardiac involvement in MPA is even more rarely described. Older cohort studies suggest a cardiac event rate between 9 and 15% but do not differentiate between vasculitic cardiac involvement from cardiac complications secondary to renal failure and a hyperinflammatory state (78).

Cardiac involvement

Pericarditis appears to be the most common clinical manifestation of cardiac disease in both GPA and MPA followed by cardiomyopathy (75,79). Valvular involvement is better described in GPA with the aortic valve being most often involved, followed by the mitral valve (80). Valvular involvement leads to leaflet thickening and dysfunction with subsequent regurgitation or stenosis. Occasionally, mass-like vegetations mimicking infective endocarditis have occurred (75). Cardiac arrhythmias, including advanced heart block, have been described more commonly in GPA, possibly owing to the granulomatous infiltrative nature of the disease. Accelerated coronary artery disease is well described in GPA patients with a two-to-four-fold relative risk compared to matched controls (81). Frank coronary arteritis is very uncommon in either GPA or MPA; however, older case reports and autopsy series have demonstrated this finding post-mortem (82).

The implications of active cardiac involvement in GPA are debated. A large North American cohort study of GPA patients found no association between cardiac involvement and a higher risk of mortality or disease relapse (75). Conversely, European cohorts have described cardiovascular involvement as a risk factor for resistance to treatment as well as for disease relapse (83). It is agreed upon that GPA patients as a whole are at higher, long-term risk for cardiovascular disease, namely ischemic heart disease, regardless of cardiac involvement in the acute setting (81). There is little data in MPA to conclude whether cardiac involvement specifically portends a worse prognosis compared to other end-organ manifestations.

Treatment

Treatment of GPA and MPA with cardiac involvement follows the same paradigm of treatment for either of these diseases with any severe end-organ manifestations. Steroids, either pulse dose or high oral dose, are recommended. Cyclophosphamide or rituximab are the main considerations in induction steroid-sparing therapy to achieve remission. Use of rituximab is supported by the RAVE trial, which demonstrated comparable efficacy of rituximab in GPA and MPA patients compared to cyclophosphamide (84). ACR/Vasculitis Foundation guidelines favor the use of rituximab over cyclophosphamide in active, severe GPA/MPA (69). Unlike in EGPA, there is no recommendation for patients with cardiac disease specifically. If remission with rituximab is achieved, this may be continued at adjusted dosing for maintenance therapy. Methotrexate and azathioprine are second-line maintenance agents. Avacopan is a novel oral c5a inhibitor approved as an adjunctive, steroid-sparing agent to induce remission in patients with severe AAV (85). Although specific cardiac outcomes with avacopan are not described, AAV patients on the therapy had significantly decreased cumulative GC exposure compared to standard therapy. Given the known risk of accelerated atherosclerosis with GC use, the use of avacopan may help mitigate long-term risk for cardiovascular disease.

CRYOGLOBULINEMIC VASCULITIS (CV)

Background/Epidemiology

Cryoglobulinemia refers to a spectrum of disease characterized by the deposition of variable immunoglobulins throughout the vasculature, which precipitate in temperatures below 37 degrees Celsius outside the body. Cryoglobulinemia is classified by the type of circulating immunoglobulin, which is often associated with underlying disease etiologies, including connective tissue disease, infection, and hematologic malignancy. Clinically significant cryoglobulinemia is rare, affecting an estimated 1 in 100,000 individuals (86).

Clinical presentation and diagnosis

Clinical presentation is variable depending on the type of immunoglobulin involved. Palpable purpura, digital ulceration and ischemia, and mononeuritis multiplex may be suggestive in the correct context. Suspicion may be raised in patients with underlying infection, including HBV, HCV, and HIV, clonal hematologic malignancies, or autoimmune disease.

Cardiac involvement

Cardiac involvement in CV is very rare and is more often seen in patients with mixed (type II) cryoglobulinemia (87). A French study of patients with monoclonal (type I) cryoglobulinemia did not describe cardiac involvement in any of these individuals (85). The overall presence of cardiac involvement appears to occur in 3–6% of patients with cryoglobulinemia of any kind (87–89). Cardiomyopathy is the most commonly described manifestation and often results in ventricular dilation (89). Post-mortem case studies have reported the presence of coronary vasculitis (90). Valvular

involvement is limited to individual patient case reports (87).

Treatment

Therapy is targeted toward any underlying-associated etiology. Antiviral agents may be used in the treatment of a CV patient with underlying hepatitis C infection. In patients with end-organ involvement, immunosuppression is often employed and most typically includes GCs and rituximab, though cyclophosphamide may be used as well. Depending on clinical severity and treatment response, plasmapheresis may be added.

BEHÇET'S SYNDROME (BS)

Background/Epidemiology

Behçet's syndrome (BS) is a variable vessel vasculitis that can affect arteries and veins of all calibers. It equally affects individuals of both genders and presents most frequently during the third or fourth decade of life. The disease is more common among individuals with ancestry along the ancient Silk Road (the prevalence in Turkey is more than 300 cases per 100,000) (91). Genetic and epigenetic factors are believed to underlie the disease, including the increased risk conferred by the HLA-B51 allele. The impairment of cell-mediated immunity and environmental factors likely also play important roles in BS (92).

Clinical features and diagnosis

Most patients have recurrent aphthous oral ulcers that are typically painful but resolve spontaneously within several weeks. Painful, scarring genital ulcerations are also a frequent symptom. Various skin manifestations have been described. Ocular lesions include uveitis (both anterior and posterior), retinal vasculitis, and optic neuritis. Neurologic, gastrointestinal, and vascular manifestations can be seen in patients with BS. When the vasculature is involved, veins and arteries of all sizes may be affected, and vascular disease is responsible for high morbidity and mortality (93). Venous thrombosis is more common in BS than arterial thrombosis. Pulmonary artery aneurysm is the most specific pulmonary manifestation to BS, not commonly occurring in other autoimmune conditions. It may mimic pulmonary embolism and result in pulmonary artery thrombosis associated with high morbidity and mortality.

Cardiac involvement

Cardiac involvement is less common in BS, though virtually any structure of the heart may be affected, including the endocardium, myocardium, pericardium, valves, coronary arteries, and aortic root. Pericarditis has been reported as the most frequent cardiac manifestation and may range in severity from asymptomatic pericardial effusion to pericardial tamponade (94). Coronary aneurysm can be seen in patients with BS who undergo angiography, some of which originally presented as acute coronary syndrome. Intracardiac thrombus has been described as a major cause of cardiac morbidity, likely due to embolization (94). Cardiomyopathy leading to systolic and/or diastolic heart failure has been described. Aortitis is frequent and may often involve the aortic root.

Treatment

The treatment of BS is organ-based. Topical therapies can be used for oral and genital ulcers. For the treatment and prevention of recurrent ulcers, colchicine or apremilast may be used. For end-organ manifestations, including cardiac disease, the initiation of GC should be strongly considered. Steroid sparing immunosuppressives, including azathioprine, calcineurin inhibitors, TNFi, and CYC, have been used (94,95). It is noteworthy that thrombosis in BS has an inflammatory basis and thus should be treated with immunosuppressive therapy. Anticoagulative therapy is controversial but can be considered depending on thrombus location, as certain lesions, such as pulmonary artery aneurysms, are at high risk for catastrophic bleeding. In general, cardiac involvement portends a worse prognosis in BS compared to those without it (95).

REFERENCES

1. Pugh D, Karabayas M, Basu N, Cid MC, Goel R, Goodyear CS, et al. Large-vessel vasculitis. Nat Rev Dis Primers. 2022;7(1):93.
2. Boes CJ. Bayard Horton's clinicopathological description of giant cell (temporal) arteritis. Cephalalgia. 2007;27(1):68–75.
3. Greigert H, Genet C, Ramon A, Bonnotte B, Samson M. New insights into the pathogenesis of giant cell arteritis: mechanisms involved in maintaining vascular inflammation. J Clin Med. 2022;11(10):2905.
4. Weyand CM, Younge BR, Goronzy JJ. IFN-gamma and IL-17: the two faces of T-cell pathology in giant cell arteritis. Curr Opin Rheumatol. 2011;23(1):43–9.
5. Hellmich B, Agueda A, Monti S, Buttgereit F, de Boysson H, Brouwer E, et al. 2018 Update of the EULAR recommendations for the management of large vessel vasculitis. Ann Rheum Dis. 2020;79(1):19–30.
6. Gonzalez-Gay MA, Barros S, Lopez-Diaz MJ, Garcia-Porrua C, Sanchez-Andrade A, Llorca J. Giant cell arteritis: disease patterns of clinical presentation in a series of 240 patients. Medicine (Baltimore). 2005;84(5):269–76.
7. Ponte C, Grayson PC, Robson JC, Suppiah R, Gribbons KB, Judge A, et al. 2022 American College of Rheumatology/EULAR classification criteria for giant cell arteritis. Arthritis Rheumatol. 2022;74(12):1881–9.
8. Tiosano S, Adler Y, Azrielant S, Yavne Y, Gendelman O, Ben-Ami Shor D, et al. Pericarditis among giant cell arteritis patients: from myth to reality. Clin Cardiol. 2018;41(5):623–7.
9. de Boysson H, Aouba A. An updated review of cardiovascular events in giant cell arteritis. J Clin Med. 2022;11(4):1005.
10. Fayyaz B, Rehman HJ. The spectrum of pericardial involvement in giant cell arteritis and polymyalgia rheumatica: a systematic review of literature. J Clin Rheumatol. 2021;27(1):5–10.
11. Udayakumar PD, Chandran AK, Crowson CS, Warrington KJ, Matteson EL. Cardiovascular risk and acute coronary syndrome in giant cell arteritis: a population-based retrospective cohort study. Arthritis Care Res (Hoboken). 2015;67(3):396–402.
12. Greigert H, Zeller M, Putot A, Steinmetz E, Terriat B, Maza M, et al. Myocardial infarction during giant cell arteritis: a cohort study. Eur J Intern Med. 2021;89:30–8.

13. Nuenninghoff DM, Hunder GG, Christianson TJ, McClelland RL, Matteson EL. Incidence and predictors of large-artery complication (aortic aneurysm, aortic dissection, and/or large-artery stenosis) in patients with giant cell arteritis: a population-based study over 50 years. Arthritis Rheum. 2003;48(12):3522–31.

14. Masood Noori MA, Mohammadian M, Saeed H, et al. Giant-Cell Aortitis-Induced Acute Aortic Insufficiency: An Underestimated Etiology. 2022;24.

15. Muratore F, Crescentini F, Spaggiari L, Pazzola G, Casali M, Boiardi L, et al. Aortic dilatation in patients with large vessel vasculitis: a longitudinal case control study using PET/CT. Semin Arthritis Rheum. 2019;48(6):1074–82.

16. de Boysson H, Daumas A, Vautier M, Parienti JJ, Liozon E, Lambert M, et al. Large-vessel involvement and aortic dilation in giant-cell arteritis. A multicenter study of 549 patients. Autoimmun Rev. 2018;17(4):391–8.

17. Maz M, Chung SA, Abril A, Langford CA, Gorelik M, Guyatt G, et al. 2021 American College of Rheumatology/ Vasculitis Foundation guideline for the management of giant cell arteritis and Takayasu arteritis. Arthritis Rheumatol. 2021;73(8):1349–65.

18. Stone JH, Tuckwell K, Dimonaco S, Klearman M, Aringer M, Blockmans D, et al. Trial of tocilizumab in giant-cell arteritis. N Engl J Med. 2017;377(4):317–28.

19. Dreyer L, Faurschou M, Baslund B. A population-based study of Takayasu's arteritis in eastern Denmark. Clin Exp Rheumatol. 2011;29(1 Suppl 64):S40–2.

20. Mohammad AJ, Mandl T. Takayasu arteritis in southern Sweden. J Rheumatol. 2015;42(5):853–8.

21. Watts R, Al-Taiar A, Mooney J, Scott D, Macgregor A. The epidemiology of Takayasu arteritis in the UK. Rheumatology (Oxford). 2009;48(8):1008–11.

22. Watanabe R, Berry GJ, Liang DH, Goronzy JJ, Weyand CM. Pathogenesis of giant cell arteritis and Takayasu arteritis-similarities and differences. Curr Rheumatol Rep. 2020;22(10):68.

23. Terao C. Revisited HLA and non-HLA genetics of Takayasu arteritis--where are we?. 2016;61(1).

24. Kumar Chauhan S, Kumar Tripathy N, Sinha N, Singh M, Nityanand S. Cellular and humoral immune responses to mycobacterial heat shock protein-65 and its human homologue in Takayasu's arteritis. Clin Exp Immunol. 2004;138(3):547–53.

25. Shingadia D, Das L, Klein-Gitelman M, Chadwick E. Takayasu's arteritis in a human immunodeficiency virus-infected adolescent. Clin Infect Dis. 1999;29(2):458–9.

26. Schmidt J, Kermani TA, Bacani AK, Crowson CS, Cooper LT, Matteson EL, et al. Diagnostic features, treatment, and outcomes of Takayasu arteritis in a US cohort of 126 patients. Mayo Clin Proc. 2013;88(8):822–30.

27. Russo RAG, Katsicas MM. Takayasu arteritis. Front Pediatr. 2018;6:265.

28. Grayson PC, Ponte C, Suppiah R, Robson JC, Gribbons KB, Judge A, et al. 2022 American College of Rheumatology/EULAR classification criteria for Takayasu arteritis. Ann Rheum Dis. 2022;81(12):1654–60.

29. Ouali S, Kacem S, Ben Fradj F, Gribaa R, Naffeti E, Remedi F, et al. Takayasu arteritis with coronary aneurysms causing acute myocardial infarction in a young man. Tex Heart Inst J. 2011;38(2):183–6.

30. Toledano K, Guralnik L, Lorber A, Ofer A, Yigla M, Rozin A, et al. Pulmonary arteries involvement in Takayasu's arteritis: two cases and literature review. Semin Arthritis Rheum. 2011;41(3):461–70.

31. Sueyoshi E, Sakamoto I, Hayashi K. Aortic aneurysms in patients with Takayasu's arteritis: CT evaluation. AJR Am J Roentgenol. 2000;175(6):1727–33.

32. Misra DP, Shenoy SN. Cardiac involvement in primary systemic vasculitis and potential drug therapies to reduce cardiovascular risk. Rheumatol Int. 2017;37(1):151–67.

33. Liang P, Hoffman GS. Advances in the medical and surgical treatment of Takayasu arteritis. Curr Opin Rheumatol. 2005;17(1):16–24.

34. Ogino H, Matsuda H, Minatoya K, Sasaki H, Tanaka H, Matsumura Y, et al. Overview of late outcome of medical and surgical treatment for Takayasu arteritis. Circulation. 2008;118(25):2738–47.

35. Holman RC, Belay ED, Christensen KY, Folkema AM, Steiner CA, Schonberger LB. Hospitalizations for Kawasaki syndrome among children in the United States, 1997–2007. Pediatr Infect Dis J. 2010;29(6):483–8.

36. Stockheim JA, Innocentini N, Shulman ST. Kawasaki disease in older children and adolescents. J Pediatr. 2000;137(2):250–2.

37. McCrindle BW, Rowley AH, Newburger JW, Burns JC, Bolger AF, Gewitz M, et al. Diagnosis, treatment, and long-term management of Kawasaki disease: a scientific statement for health professionals from the American Heart Association. Circulation. 2017;135(17):e927–e99.

38. Du ZD, Zhao D, Du J, Zhang YL, Lin Y, Liu C, et al. Epidemiologic study on Kawasaki disease in Beijing from 2000 through 2004. Pediatr Infect Dis J. 2007;26(5):449–51.

39. Nakamura Y, Yashiro M, Uehara R, Sadakane A, Chihara I, Aoyama Y, et al. Epidemiologic features of Kawasaki disease in Japan: results of the 2007–2008 nationwide survey. J Epidemiol. 2010;20(4):302–7.

40. Park YW, Han JW, Hong YM, Ma JS, Cha SH, Kwon TC, et al. Epidemiological features of Kawasaki disease in Korea, 2006–2008. Pediatr Int. 2011;53(1):36–9.

41. Holman RC, Christensen KY, Belay ED, Steiner CA, Effler PV, Miyamura J, et al. Racial/ethnic differences in the incidence of Kawasaki syndrome among children in Hawaii. Hawaii Med J. 2010;69(8):194–7.

42. Burns JC, Herzog L, Fabri O, Tremoulet AH, Rodo X, Uehara R, et al. Seasonality of Kawasaki disease: a global perspective. PLOS ONE. 2013;8(9):e74529.

43. Cai Z, Zuo R, Liu Y. Characteristics of Kawasaki disease in older children. Clin Pediatr (Phila). 2011;50(10):952–6.

44. Bratincsak A, Reddy VD, Purohit PJ, Tremoulet AH, Molkara DP, Frazer JR, et al. Coronary artery dilation in acute Kawasaki disease and acute illnesses associated with fever. Pediatr Infect Dis J. 2012;31(9):924–6.

45. Kao CH, Hsieh KS, Wang YL, Wang SJ, Yeh SH. The detection of ventricular dysfunction and carditis in children with Kawasaki disease using equilibrium multigated blood pooling ventriculography and 99Tcm-HMPAO-labelled WBC heart scans. Nucl Med Commun. 1993;14(7):539–43.

46. Harada M, Yokouchi Y, Oharaseki T, Matsui K, Tobayama H, Tanaka N, et al. Histopathological characteristics of myocarditis in acute-phase Kawasaki disease. Histopathology. 2012;61(6):1156–67.

47. Printz BF, Sleeper LA, Newburger JW, Minich LL, Bradley T, Cohen MS, et al. Noncoronary cardiac abnormalities are associated with coronary artery dilation and with laboratory inflammatory markers in acute Kawasaki disease. J Am Coll Cardiol. 2011;57(1):86–92.

48. Gidding SS, Shulman ST, Ilbawi M, Crussi F, Duffy CE. Mucocutaneous lymph node syndrome (Kawasaki disease): delayed aortic and mitral insufficiency secondary to active valvulitis. J Am Coll Cardiol. 1986;7(4):894–7.

49. Mori M, Miyamae T, Imagawa T, Katakura S, Kimura K, Yokota S. Meta-analysis of the results of intravenous gamma globulin treatment of coronary artery lesions in Kawasaki disease. Mod Rheumatol. 2004;14(5):361–6.

50. Murphy DJ Jr., Huhta JC. Treatment of Kawasaki syndrome with intravenous gamma globulin. N Engl J Med. 1987;316(14):881.

51. Oates-Whitehead RM, Baumer JH, Haines L, Love S, Maconochie IK, Gupta A, et al. Intravenous immunoglobulin for the treatment of Kawasaki disease in children. Cochrane Database Syst Rev. 2003;2003(4):CD004000.

52. Kobayashi T, Saji T, Otani T, Takeuchi K, Nakamura T, Arakawa H, et al. Efficacy of immunoglobulin plus prednisolone for prevention of coronary artery abnormalities in severe Kawasaki disease (RAISE study): a randomised, open-label, blinded-endpoints trial. Lancet. 2012;379(9826):1613–20.

53. Newburger JW, Takahashi M, Burns JC. Kawasaki disease. J Am Coll Cardiol. 2016;67(14):1738–49.

54. Tremoulet AH, Jain S, Jaggi P, Jimenez-Fernandez S, Pancheri JM, Sun X, et al. Infliximab for intensification of primary therapy for Kawasaki disease: a phase 3 randomised, double-blind, placebo-controlled trial. Lancet. 2014;383(9930):1731–8.

55. Watts RA, Lane SE, Scott DG, Koldingsnes W, Nossent H, Gonzalez-Gay MA, et al. Epidemiology of vasculitis in Europe. Ann Rheum Dis. 2001;60(12):1156–7.

56. Watts RA, Scott DG. Epidemiology of the vasculitides. Semin Respir Crit Care Med. 2004;25(5):455–64.

57. Holsinger DR, Osmundson PJ, Edwards JE. The heart in periarteritis nodosa. Circulation. 1962;25:610–8.

58. Schrader ML, Hochman JS, Bulkley BH. The heart in polyarteritis nodosa: a clinicopathologic study. Am Heart J. 1985;109(6):1353–9.

59. Lai J, Zhao L, Zhong H, Zhou J, Guo X, Xu D, et al. Characteristics and outcomes of coronary artery involvement in polyarteritis nodosa. Can J Cardiol. 2021;37(6):895–903.

60. Bourgarit A, Toumelin PL, Pagnoux C, Cohen P, Mahr A, Guern VL, et al. Deaths occurring during the first year after treatment onset for polyarteritis nodosa, microscopic polyangiitis, and Churg-Strauss syndrome: a retrospective analysis of causes and factors predictive of mortality based on 595 patients. Medicine (Baltimore). 2005;84(5):323–30.

61. Gayraud M, Guillevin L, le Toumelin P, Cohen P, Lhote F, Casassus P, et al. Long-term follow-up of polyarteritis nodosa, microscopic polyangiitis, and Churg-Strauss syndrome: analysis of four prospective trials including 278 patients. Arthritis Rheum. 2001;44(3):666–75.

62. Chung SA, Gorelik M, Langford CA, Maz M, Abril A, Guyatt G, et al. 2021 American College of Rheumatology/Vasculitis Foundation guideline for the management of polyarteritis nodosa. Arthritis Care Res (Hoboken). 2021;73(8):1061–70.

63. Jakes RW, Kwon N, Nordstrom B, Goulding R, Fahrbach K, Tarpey J, et al. Burden of illness associated with eosinophilic granulomatosis with polyangiitis: a systematic literature review and meta-analysis. Clin Rheumatol. 2021;40(12):4829–36.

64. Pakbaz M, Pakbaz M. Cardiac involvement in eosinophilic granulomatosis with polyangiitis: a meta-analysis of 62 case reports. J Tehran Heart Cent. 2020;15(1):18–26.

65. Neumann T, Manger B, Schmid M, Kroegel C, Hansch A, Kaiser WA, et al. Cardiac involvement in Churg-Strauss syndrome: impact of endomyocarditis. Medicine (Baltimore). 2009;88(4):236–43.

66. Liu S, Guo L, Zhang Z, Li M, Zeng X, Wang L, et al. Cardiac manifestations of eosinophilic granulomatosis with polyangiitis from a single-center cohort in China: clinical features and associated factors. Ther Adv Chronic Dis. 2021;12. doi:2040622320987051.

67. Garcia-Vives E, Rodriguez-Palomares JF, Harty L, Solans-Laque R, Jayne D. Heart disease in eosinophilic granulomatosis with polyangiitis (EGPA) patients: a screening approach proposal. Rheumatology (Oxford). 2021;60(10):4538–47.

68. Springer JM, Kalot MA, Husainat NM, Byram KW, Dua AB, James KE, et al. Eosinophilic granulomatosis with polyangiitis: a systematic review and meta-analysis of test accuracy and benefits and harms of common treatments. ACR Open Rheumatol. 2021;3(2):101–10.

69. Chung SA, Langford CA, Maz M, Abril A, Gorelik M, Guyatt G, et al. 2021 American College of Rheumatology/Vasculitis Foundation guideline for the management of antineutrophil cytoplasmic antibody-associated vasculitis. Arthritis Rheumatol. 2021;73(8):1366–83.

70. Terrier B, Pugnet G, de Moreuil C, Bonnotte B, Benhamou Y, Diot E, et al. Rituximab versus conventional therapeutic strategy for remission induction in eosinophilic granulomatosis with polyangiitis: a double-blind, randomized, controlled trial [Abstract]. Arthritis Rheumatol. 2021;73 (suppl 9) doi.org/10.1002/art.41966

71. Wechsler ME, Akuthota P, Jayne D, Khoury P, Klion A, Langford CA, et al. Mepolizumab or placebo for eosinophilic granulomatosis with polyangiitis. N Engl J Med. 2017;376(20):1921–32.

72. Hellmich B, Sanchez-Alamo B, Schirmer JH, Berti A, Blockmans D, Cid MC, et al. EULAR recommendations for the management of ANCA-associated vasculitis: 2022 update. Ann Rheum Dis. 2024;83(1):30–47.

73. Berti A, Cornec D, Crowson CS, Specks U, Matteson EL. The epidemiology of antineutrophil cytoplasmic autoantibody-associated vasculitis in Olmsted County, Minnesota: a twenty-year US population-based study. Arthritis Rheumatol. 2017;69(12):2338–50.

74. Koldingsnes W, Nossent JC. Baseline features and initial treatment as predictors of remission and relapse in Wegener's granulomatosis. J Rheumatol. 2003;30(1):80–8.

75. McGeoch L, Carette S, Cuthbertson D, Hoffman GS, Khalidi N, Koening CL, et al. Cardiac involvement in granulomatosis with polyangiitis. J Rheumatol. 2015;42(7):1209–12.

76. Al-Mehisen R, Alnemri K, Al-Mohaissen M. Cardiac imaging of a patient with unusual presentation of granulomatosis with polyangiitis: a case report and review of the literature. J Nucl Cardiol. 2021;28(2):441–55.

77. Hazebroek MR, Kemna MJ, Schalla S, Sanders-van Wijk S, Gerretsen SC, Dennert R, et al. Prevalence and prognostic relevance of cardiac involvement in ANCA-associated vasculitis: eosinophilic granulomatosis with polyangiitis and granulomatosis with polyangiitis. Int J Cardiol. 2015;199:170–9.

78. Guillevin L, Durand-Gasselin B, Cevallos R, Gayraud M, Lhote F, Callard P, et al. Microscopic polyangiitis: clinical and laboratory findings in eighty-five patients. Arthritis Rheum. 1999;42(3):421–30.

79. Knockaert DC. Cardiac involvement in systemic inflammatory diseases. Eur Heart J. 2007;28(15):1797–804.

80. Miloslavsky E, Unizony S. The heart in vasculitis. Rheum Dis Clin North Am. 2014;40(1):11–26.

81. Mourguet M, Chauveau D, Faguer S, Ruidavets JB, Bejot Y, Ribes D, et al. Increased ischemic stroke, acute coronary artery disease and mortality in patients with granulomatosis with polyangiitis and microscopic polyangiitis. J Autoimmun. 2019;96:134–41.

82. Dewan R, Bittar H, Lacomis J, Ocak I. Granulomatosis with polyangiitis presenting with coronary artery and pericardial involvement. Case Rep Radiol. 2015;2015:516437.

83. Walsh M, Flossmann O, Berden A, Westman K, Hoglund P, Stegeman C, et al. Risk factors for relapse of antineutrophil cytoplasmic antibody-associated vasculitis. Arthritis Rheum. 2012;64(2):542–8.

84. Stone JH, Merkel PA, Spiera R, Seo P, Langford CA, Hoffman GS, et al. Rituximab versus cyclophosphamide for ANCA-associated vasculitis. N Engl J Med. 2010;363(3):221–32.

85. Jayne DRW, Merkel PA, Schall TJ, Bekker P, Group AS. Avacopan for the treatment of ANCA-associated vasculitis. N Engl J Med. 2021;384(7):599–609.

86. Silva F, Pinto C, Barbosa A, Borges T, Dias C, Almeida J. New insights in cryoglobulinemic vasculitis. J Autoimmun. 2019;105:102313.

87. He K, Zhang Y, Wang W, Wang Y, Sha Y, Zeng X. Clinical characteristics of cryoglobulinemia with cardiac involvement in a single center. Front Cardiovasc Med. 2021;8:744648.

88. Terrier B, Karras A, Kahn JE, Le Guenno G, Marie I, Benarous L, et al. The spectrum of type I cryoglobulinemia vasculitis: new insights based on 64 cases. Medicine (Baltimore). 2013;92(2):61–8.

89. Terrier B, Karras A, Cluzel P, Collet JP, Sene D, Saadoun D, et al. Presentation and prognosis of cardiac involvement in hepatitis C virus-related vasculitis. Am J Cardiol. 2013;111(2):265–72.

90. Maestroni A, Caviglia AG, Colzani M, Borghi A, Monti G, Picozzi G, et al. Heart involvement in essential mixed cryoglobulinemia. Ric Clin Lab. 1986;16(2):381–3.

91. Yazici Y, Hatemi G, Bodaghi B, Cheon JH, Suzuki N, Ambrose N, et al. Behcet syndrome. Nat Rev Dis Primers. 2021;7(1):67.

92. Takeuchi M, Ombrello MJ, Kirino Y, Erer B, Tugal-Tutkun I, Seyahi E, et al. A single endoplasmic reticulum aminopeptidase-1

protein allotype is a strong risk factor for Behcet's disease in HLA-B*51 carriers. Ann Rheum Dis. 2016;75(12):2208–11.

93. Saadoun D, Asli B, Wechsler B, Houman H, Geri G, Desseaux K, et al. Long-term outcome of arterial lesions in Behcet disease: a series of 101 patients. Medicine (Baltimore). 2012;91(1):18–24.

94. Demirelli S, Degirmenci H, Inci S, Arisoy A. Cardiac manifestations in Behcet's disease. Intractable Rare Dis Res. 2015;4(2):70–5.

95. Alpsoy E, Leccese P, Emmi G, Ohno S. Treatment of Behcet's disease: an algorithmic multidisciplinary approach. Front Med (Lausanne). 2021;8:624795.

12

Preventive cardiac health for the rheumatologist

ALAA DIAB, BREANNA HANSEN, DIANA H. TRAN,
JESSICA N. HOLTZMAN, AND MARTHA GULATI

INTRODUCTION

Autoimmune rheumatic diseases (ARDs) are systemic inflammatory diseases that affect the cardiovascular system in varying degrees.[1] Cardiac involvement includes the vasculature, myocardium, pericardium, valves, and the conduction system, which can present silently or lead to critical conditions with high morbidity and mortality.[1-3] The risk of cardiovascular disease (CVD) in this population is increased due to the high prevalence of traditional atherosclerotic CVD (ASCVD) risk factors like diabetes, hypertension, and kidney disease, as well as the inflammatory process of the disease itself, with pro-thrombotic state, cytokines, and antibodies contributing to accelerated atherosclerosis formation. Furthermore, the medications used in the management course can have varying effects on the cardiovascular system, which may contribute to the development and progression of ASCVD.[4]

Given the high morbidity and mortality of ASCVD in the ARD population, primary and secondary prevention are key components in the care of these patients. Primary prevention constitutes of appropriate screening early in the disease before any cardiac manifestations are present. This includes using atherosclerosis risk-specific calculators, different imaging modalities, adjustment of the medical management, and other blood tests like lipid profile screening. Secondary prevention entails medical management for specific cardiovascular manifestations along with continued imaging for disease progress tracking. Although collaborations between the rheumatologist and cardiologist are common, they often happen in the secondary and tertiary prevention stages rather than primary. The underrecognized need for early intervention contributes to the increased ASCVD burden.

There are many barriers to ASCVD prevention in the ARD population, including inadequate or delayed screening, undertreatment of traditional risk factors, and not taking into consideration ASCVD risk and burden in the clinical care and treatment choices, in addition to risk underestimation. For patients, often there are varying health literacy levels that can contribute further to a lack of understanding of this important clinical association. Lastly, research is quite limited in this area, with most data regarding the risk of ARDs to ASCVD being retrospective or observational. All these barriers can be addressed mostly with early collaboration between the rheumatologist and cardiologist, utilizing risk ASCVD scores, and educating the ARD population early on about the ASCVD risks, particularly the modifiable ones.

In this chapter, we examine the cardiac manifestations of ARDs as well as the primary and

DOI: 10.1201/9781003386711-12

secondary prevention of ASCVD in this population, including the limitations and barriers to their cardiac care.

EPIDEMIOLOGY

ASCVD is common in patients with ARDs.[5] In an analysis of data from a single center, the prevalence of ASCVD was 29.7% and 14.7% for Black and White adults with ARDs, respectively.[6] The prevalence of ASCVD in patients with systemic lupus erythematosus (SLE) was 25.6%, while in those without SLE it was 19.2% in a study of 252,676 patients with SLE and 758,034 matched patients without SLE.[7] Furthermore, women of ages 35–44 with SLE are more than 50 times more likely to have a myocardial infarction (MI) compared to women of similar age without SLE.[8] In patients with rheumatoid arthritis (RA), there is a 1.5- to 2-fold increased risk of developing ASCVD compared to the general population, where ASCVD is found to be the leading cause of death.[8,9] In addition, RA is associated with higher rates of MI in women and with higher rates of all-cause mortality and vascular events compared to patients without RA or with osteoarthritis.[10,11] Furthermore, psoriatic arthritis (PsA) was found to be an independent risk factor for increased incidence of ASCVD, where patients with more severe psoriatic disease activity experience higher rates of MI.[12,13] On the other hand, studies on ankylosing spondylitis remain controversial, as some showed no difference in ASCVD mortality from the general population, while others showed an increased risk.[13,14]

CARDIOVASCULAR MANIFESTATIONS OF ARDs

The cardiovascular manifestations of ARDs are a prominent source of morbidity and mortality for patients diagnosed with systemic inflammatory conditions.[15] Much remains unknown about the cardiovascular manifestations of these conditions and the underlying pathophysiology. The cardiovascular effects of ARDs include accelerated atherosclerosis, valvular disease, pericardial disease, myocardial disease, and disorders of the electrical conduction system.[16] Further, cardiac manifestations may arise both from the primary disease states and the associated treatment modalities.[17]

Early recognition of the potential cardiovascular complications of rheumatologic disease is essential to allow for aggressive primary and secondary preventative management of risk factors, as well as proactive treatment of inflammatory rheumatologic conditions. While the focus of this chapter is ASCVD in the ARD population, recognizing and managing other cardiac manifestations can help decrease CVD burden in general.

Accelerated atherosclerosis

Patients with chronic, systemic inflammatory disorders have been demonstrated to experience accelerated atherosclerosis and excess mortality due to coronary artery disease (CAD). A large meta-analysis estimated that over 50% of excess mortality in patients with RA is due to CVD; similarly, CVD is reported as the leading cause of mortality among patients with SLE.[18] Accelerated atherosclerosis and resultant CAD contribute significantly to cardiovascular mortality in this patient population.

Though the exact mechanism remains unknown, chronic inflammation contributes to premature atherosclerosis by a variety of mechanisms.[19,20] Chronic inflammatory conditions may be associated with elevated rates of traditional cardiovascular risk factors, such as hypertension, dyslipidemia, and obesity.[21] Additionally, ARDs may result in mobility limitation and place patients at risk for reduced physical activity and lower physical fitness as compared to those without ARD.[22,23] However, beyond traditional ASCVD risk factors, it has been suggested that pro-inflammatory cytokines, including TNF-alpha and interleukin-6, result in endothelial dysfunction and activation, allowing for leukocyte infiltration.[24] An inflammatory milieu has also been associated with traditional ASCVD, including dyslipidemia and increased insulin resistance.[18] Other rheumatic conditions, like systemic sclerosis (SSc), have also been shown to be associated with microvascular involvement that may ultimately increase risk for myocardial dysfunction and ASCVD as well.[25]

Valvular, pericardial, and myocardial disease

The protean effects of autoimmune disease on the cardiovascular system extend to the cardiac valves, pericardium, and myocardium. Among patients with RA, mitral regurgitation is the most common valvular lesion seen, whereas in patients with SLE, Libman-Sacks vegetations or nonbacterial endocarditis are more common.[15] Patients with ankylosing spondylitis have been found to have markedly elevated rates of aortic root thickening and aortic regurgitation as compared to age-matched controls, with one study finding 80% of patients with ankylosing spondylitis to have aortic root or valvular disease on transesophageal echocardiography.[26]

Both systolic and diastolic heart failure are seen at increased rates in patients with RA, SLE, and SSc.[27–30] Pericardial disease is most notably associated with SLE, manifesting as pericarditis or pericardial effusion. Pericardial disease is seen to a lesser extent in RA and SSc and is most often detected only on autopsy.[15,16,30]

Electrical conduction

Conduction disease is a common manifestation of ARDs, including SLE, RA, and SSc.[31] The prominent electrical disturbances concord with the underlying pathophysiology by disease state, resulting in accelerated atherosclerosis, vasculitis, thrombosis, or fibrosis of the myocardium and conduction system.

Patients with RA have a markedly increased risk of CAD, which predisposes them to sudden cardiac death and ventricular arrhythmias.[15] One study found an increased rate of cardiac involvement with nodular as compared to non-nodular RA (71.9% vs 42.9%) defined by echocardiography, 24-hour Holter monitor, and resting ECG.[32] However, the authors reported no difference between the groups in arrhythmia burden, despite more patients with 1 mm ST depressions in the nodular RA group.[32]

In patients with SLE, the most commonly reported arrhythmias include sinus tachycardia, atrial fibrillation, and ectopic atrial beats, which may recede with treatment of the underlying disease state. Further, in neonatal lupus, approximately 3% of infants will develop complete heart block.[33] Treatment effects should be noted, as well. For instance, hydroxychloroquine has been associated with QT-interval prolongation and sinus bradycardia.[15]

In SSc, studies suggest that as many as 30% of patients may experience supraventricular tachycardias related to myocardial fibrosis.[34,35] There has also been a suggestion of increased rates of ventricular arrhythmias, including premature ventricular beats, as compared to controls.[34,35]

Though the treatment of arrhythmias associated with autoimmune disease does not differ from that of patients without autoimmune disease, care team members should maintain a high index of suspicion for arrhythmia and subsequent referral to a cardiologist in this patient population.

RISK FACTORS FOR ASCVD

Traditional risk factors for ASCVD

Traditional risk factors for ASCVD include smoking, hypertension, hypercholesterolemia, and diabetes. Other well-known risk factors include insulin resistance, obesity, a family history of CVD, and peripheral vascular disease (PVD). Social determinants of health and psychosocial factors also play a key role in the risk of developing ASCVD. Patients with ARD have an increased prevalence of traditional risk factors as well as having independent disease-specific risk factors, as outlined below. Given their increased risk, they are to be considered a risk-enhancing feature for ASCVD risk calculations. Not only do these autoimmune disorders increase the risk for CVD in general, but medications commonly used to treat these disorders also confer an increased risk. The use of corticosteroids, non-steroidal anti-inflammatory drugs (NSAIDs), including cyclooxygenase inhibitors, is associated with twice as much increased cardiovascular risk, including CHD and heart failure.[36]

SMOKING

Smoking, one of the most common modifiable risk factors for ASCVD, results in an increased and accelerated incidence of ASCVD and death by more than 50%, with the risk increasing both with the number of cigarettes consumed and with the increasing age of patients with ARDs.[37,38] Women who smoke exhibit higher morbidity and mortality from ASCVD compared to males.[38] Smoking is associated with an increased development of RA, specifically seropositive RA, and worse prognosis in both RA and SLE.[39,40]

HYPERTENSION

Hypertension, or high blood pressure, defined as a systolic blood pressure >130 mmHg or a diastolic blood pressure >80 mmHg, affects nearly half of Americans and contributes to more cardiovascular-related deaths than any of the other major modifiable cardiovascular risk factors.[41] Risk factors for developing hypertension include age, diet, physical inactivity, obesity, tobacco use, obstructive sleep apnea, family history of hypertension, socioeconomic status, and psychosocial stressors.[42] Those with ARD not only have a higher prevalence of hypertension but are also more likely to be on medications, such as COX-inhibitors, NSAIDs, and glucocorticoids, which can increase blood pressure.[43]

DIABETES

Diabetes, a well-known risk factor for ASCVD, can result in two- to eightfold higher rates of future cardiovascular events compared with nondiabetic patients.[44] Individuals with diabetes have a greater burden of additional risk factors, including hypertension, obesity, and hyperlipidemia. Moreover, diabetes presents specific cardiovascular risk enhancers, including a long duration of diabetes, nephropathy, albuminuria ≥30 μg albumin/mg creatinine, retinopathy, neuropathy, and an ankle-brachial index (ABI) <0.9.[45,46] Furthermore, hyperglycemia and insulin resistance prior to the onset of diabetes have also been suggested to increase the risk of a cardiovascular event.[47] Both diabetes and insulin resistance are known to be independent risk factors for the development of ASCVD. The prevalence of metabolic syndrome among RA patients ranges from 44% to 53%, and for SLE patients, it ranges from 16% to 32.4%.[48] Insulin resistance is particularly common in patients with SLE, RA, and ankylosing spondylitis, affecting almost half of patients.[49] This is thought to likely be secondary to inflammatory mediators, decreased physical activity, and medications such as glucocorticoids.[49]

HYPERLIPIDEMIA

Lipids typically include cholesterol levels, lipoproteins, chylomicrons, very low-density lipoprotein (VLDL), low-density lipoprotein (LDL), triglycerides (TG), apolipoproteins, and high-density lipoprotein (HDL). Hyperlipidemia, specifically LDL levels greater than the 90th percentile compared to the general population, is a major predisposing risk factor for ASCVD.[50] Hyperlipidemia can be broken down into primary and secondary causes. Secondary causes of elevated LDL commonly include diets high in saturated fats, physical inactivity, advancing age, and family history. However, certain medical conditions can cause hyperlipidemia, including hypothyroidism, diabetes, Cushing's nephrotic syndrome, and liver disease. Medications, such as thiazide diuretics, beta blockers, estrogens, corticosteroids, and antiretrovirals, can also increase LDL.[51] Although screening guidelines vary by organization, the ACC/AHA recommends initiating screening at 20 years old with repeat screening every 5 years. Screening can begin at less than 20 years old if a family history of ASCVD is present. Lipid-specific risk enhancers also exist and include lipoprotein A (Lp(a)) and ApoB. Lp(a) is transmitted strongly within families and should be checked if there is a family history of hyperlipidemia or ASCVD. Hyperlipidemia tends to occur more frequently in patients with ARD, specifically RA, PsA, ankylosing spondylitis, and SLE. Along with other markers of inflammation, individuals with SLE and RA have higher levels of oxidized-LDL, which is associated with accelerated atherosclerosis.[52,53] Active SLE is associated with higher levels of VLDL cholesterol and TGs and lower HDL.[54] Many ARD patients also receive chronic steroid therapy, which is associated with increased levels of LDL and TGs.[55] An important paradox, known as "lipid paradox", occurs in individuals with RA in which inflammation caused by active disease is associated with lower levels of LDL cholesterol but increased ASCVD.[56]

OBESITY

Obesity, defined as a BMI >30, affects nearly half the United States population and has been shown to have a linear relationship between higher BMI and the risk of CVD in general.[57] However, BMI does not consistently predict CVD, and some authors have described better outcomes in overweight and obese patients, termed the "obesity paradox".[58] This paradox is often seen in those with RA, in which an increased risk of CV death is seen in those with a lower BMI.[59] Furthermore, studies have shown that BMI does not adequately predict CV risk in women.[60] Given that ARD disproportionately effects women, it is important to take into consideration other methods of measuring fat deposition, such as waist-hip ratio, waist circumference or imaging-guided measurements of visceral adipose tissue.

FAMILY HISTORY

A pertinent family history, including the development of ASCVD or death secondary to CVD in a first-degree relative, increases the patient's risk for developing ASCVD.[61] This risk is increased when family history is considered premature, as in males <55 or females <65, and multiple family members are affected.[62]

SOCIAL DETERMINANTS OF HEALTH

Psychosocial factors, such as depression, anxiety, chronic stress, and social isolation, contribute to the development of ASCVD and are highly prevalent in patients with ARD.[63] In SLE, more severe disease is associated with lower income and educational level, disadvantaged neighborhoods, and lower social support.[64] In RA, social isolation and depression are associated with worse disease activity, while socioeconomic status is also associated with other cardiovascular risk factors, such as smoking, BMI, and diabetes.[63,64]

PERIPHERAL VASCULAR DISEASE (PVD)

PVD affects millions of people globally and increases the risk for future ASCVD. Studies have suggested that the more vascular areas affected (legs, heart, brain) are associated with a higher risk of ASCVD events.[65] Studies to date have shown an increased prevalence of PVD in patients with RA, Gout, SSc, polymyalgia rheumatica, and Bechet's.[66–70]

PRIMARY AND SECONDARY PREVENTION OF CVD

There are limited guidelines for directing clinicians on specifics of ASCVD prevention in the ARD population. Although ARDs are considered risk enhancers of ASCVD, some studies have suggested applying secondary prevention guidelines for this population prior to ASCVD manifestation. Nevertheless, primary prevention, when practiced, entails screening using risk-prediction scores, biomarkers, and imaging techniques, with the choice of specific ARDs medications being more cardioprotective than others. Figure 12.1 and Figure 12.2 provide guidance on strategies for primary and secondary prevention of ASCVD, respectively.

Risk scores

The European League Against Rheumatism (EULAR) Task Force reviewed risk scores to help establish a baseline screening guideline for clinicians and found multiple risk scores to be helpful in the primary prevention of ASCVD.[71] Many of the risk scores discussed are not ARD-specific, such as the Framingham risk score, SCORE2 chart, and the Reynolds risk score, although they include CRP as a risk factor. Nevertheless, the use of multiplication factors on top of traditional ASCVD risk score assessments was recommended by EULAR, where multiplying the Framingham risk score by a factor of 1.5 when being used for patients with RA can give a good estimate of ASCVD risk in this population.[71] On the other hand, the 2019 ACC/AHA guidelines on primary prevention of CVD were updated to include inflammatory conditions, including RA and SLE, as risk-enhancing factors.[72] One of the ARD-specific tools is QRISK®3, which was developed and used in the UK. It estimates an individual's risk of developing an MI or stroke within 10 years and includes SLE and RA in the calculation as risk factors.[73] The common features amongst all risk estimations are the traditional risk factors of age, sex, blood pressure, cholesterol, and the presence or absence of diabetes.

Imaging modalities

Several imaging modalities can be used for CVD risk assessment in ARDs. Echocardiography (ECHO) is an imaging modality for the assessment of cardiac structure and function that is widely available, inexpensive, and non-invasive.[74] It can detect subclinical cardiac manifestations, such as left ventricular diastolic dysfunction and valvular abnormalities that are prevalent in the ARD population, and can indicate the presence of ischemic disease.[74] It can also be used to monitor disease progression in those identified to have cardiac abnormalities. Furthermore, speckle-tracking echocardiography and 3-dimensional US are found to be diagnostically more accurate and can be used instead.[74] Carotid ultrasonography is another widely used modality that can be used as a non-invasive imaging technique for early detection of atherosclerotic carotid plaques and hence prediction of ASCVD, which was deemed equivalent to having CVD in the 2012 ESC guidelines. Furthermore, common carotid intima-media thickness in RA patients can be a useful indicator of atherosclerosis formation and cardiovascular events if increased.[75] Using a combination of those non-invasive ultrasonography techniques along with risk scores for primary prevention in ARDs can improve ASCVD risk stratification.[74,75]

As discussed earlier, ASCVD is one of the leading causes of death in patients with ARDs, urging the need for prevention, early detection, and management. One of the non-invasive tools used for ASCVD assessment is calculating the coronary artery calcium (CAC) score using cardiac computed tomography. It measures the amount of calcified plaque in coronary arteries to assess the risk of major cardiac events even in the asymptomatic, making it a cost-effective primary prevention modality in the ARD population.[76,77] CAC score can be used to screen RA patients with intermediate ASCVD risk, especially when screening for silent MI, as it can detect early asymptomatic CAC.[78] Furthermore, the presence of CAC in asymptomatic RA patients was associated with a 1.6-fold increase in arterial hypertension compared with patients without CAC.[79] CAC has shown effectiveness in risk assessment and treatment allocation for ASCVD primary prevention.[80]

Biomarkers

Several biomarkers have been used as a risk assessment tool for ASCVD in ARDs as well, including but not limited to inflammation markers, genetic factors, endothelial function, and immunological markers. For example, several studies explored the inflammatory modulator Interleukin-6 (IL-6) relationship with MI, where it was found to predict major recurrent cardiovascular events in patients with CAD and was used as a marker of poor prognosis in acute coronary syndrome (ACS).[81,82] High-sensitivity C-reactive protein (hs-CRP), on the other hand, is produced in the liver in response to IL-6. Thus, hs-CRP can be a simple downstream marker of IL-6 activation, and an elevated level can indicate atherosclerosis acceleration.[83] The heart failure marker, brain natriuretic peptide (BNP), has been linked to cardiovascular events and increased all-cause mortality in general.[84] According to the 2022 AHA/ACC/HFSA, BNP can be used to screen for heart failure, classifying patients with stage B at risk for heart failure if BNP is elevated with the presence of cardiac risk factors.[85] Nevertheless, it was found to

be not reliable in patients with ARDs, given the lack of correlation between BNP and cardiac dysfunction in patients with ARDs in comparison to the general population.[86] Other studies are being done on novel biomarkers such as the cytokine receptor osteoprotegerin, as it has been correlated with the presence of ASCVD in the RA population.[87,88] Another endothelial function biomarker, angiopoietin, has been associated with ASCVD in RA patients as well.[89] To date, none of these biomarkers examined in ARDs have been established to be routinely used to screen for ASCVD.

Medications

Pharmacological and nonpharmacological management of ASCVD risk factors can be used for primary and secondary prevention in ARDs. Statins, for example, have been proven effective in lowering total cholesterol and significantly improving all-cause mortality in people with ARDs by not only lowering cholesterol levels but also due to their anti-inflammatory effects.[90] For blood pressure management, angiotensin-converting enzyme inhibitors and angiotensin II blockers are the preferred agents, given their effects on inflammatory markers and endothelial function as well.[71]

ARD-specific medications have different effects on cardiac function as well as disease development and progression (Table 12.1). DMARDs, such as MTX and sulfasalazine, can have direct anti-inflammatory effects, promote reverse cholesterol transport, and inhibit foam cell formation, all of which help in ASCVD prevention directly.[91,92] Furthermore, it can have indirect effects given that it improves the overall rheumatic disease, allowing patients to be more physically active. Antimalarial medications, like hydroxychloroquine, have been associated with better CV outcomes, mainly by improving glycated hemoglobin in patients with diabetes through enhancing glycemic control in RA patients.[93] These may also be associated with improved lipid profiles in this population.[94] On the other hand, there have been no established benefits for the use of glucocorticoids for ASCVD prevention, although they are well-known anti-inflammatory agents. It is currently recommended to use the lowest dose of glucocorticoids for the shortest period possible when bridging DMARDs.[4,71,95] The evidence on biologics therapy and ASCVD prevention is controversial and inconclusive.

Table 12.1 Autoimmune rheumatic disease medications and cardiovascular effects

Class	Medication Name	MOA	CVD effect	Prevention
NSAIDs	Celecoxib, Ibuprofen, Meloxicam, Naproxen, Rofecoxib, Etocoxib	Inhibit COX activity and reduce prostaglandin synthesis	Greater COX-1 inhibition yields greater COX-2 inhibition and cardiovascular risk. Compared to placebo, Rofecoxib has the highest risk of MI, Etocoxib of vascular death, and ibuprofen of stroke. Naproxen has a lower risk of CVD events	Low-dose selective COX-1 inhibitors, i.e. aspirin, have cardiovascular protection through thrombosis prevention. However, taking a large dose of these drugs for a long time can inhibit thrombin synthesis and increase bleeding tendency
Steroids	Prednisone	Triggers apoptosis of Th¹ cells, reducing IFN-γ production by T cells, and downstream reduced systemic inflammation	Increased exposure to GCs increases the risk of CVD by causing changes in blood lipid levels, insulin resistance, diabetes, hypertension, and obesity	All CVD factors must be monitored and managed accordingly while on GC
Conventional DMARDs	Methotrexate (MTX)	Immunosuppressant and competitively inhibits dihydrofolate reductase	Reduces atherosclerosis, CVD mortality and delay the risk by 3–4 years in patients with RA, as well as reduced RR of MI	Folate supplementation is crucial
	Leflunomide	Immunomodulator with antiproliferative activities; can inhibit tyrosine kinase and LDH and interfere with pyrimidine synthesis (lymphocyte activation)	Decreases myocardial hypertrophy and prevents cardiac fibrosis but can cause hypertension	Monitor blood pressure
	Hydroxychloroquine	Antimalarial drug that interferes with lysosomal activity and autophagy.	Known to have vascular protective effects, but long-term use can rarely cause cardiac complications.	Monitor with routine EKGs and echocardiography

	Mechanism	CVD effect	Recommendation
Sulfasalazine (SSZ)	Affects absorption and metabolism of folic acid, inhibits chemotaxis of leukocytes and the activity of proteolytic enzymes, as well as inhibits NF-κB and TNF-α	Decreased CVD by improving blood lipid levels, controlling endothelial dysfunction, inhibiting platelet aggregation, and preventing carotid artery remodeling induced by inflammation	Evaluate and monitor CVD risk factors, including blood pressure and early imaging for atherosclerosis
Cyclosporine	Inhibits the response of activated T cells to IL-2 in vitro	Reduces intima-media thickness and plaque prevalence and prevents myocardial hypertrophy. It can increase blood pressure and endothelial injury	
Azathioprine (AZA)	Non-specific immunosuppressive agent formed by substituting methyl imidazole for hydrogen and sulfur atoms in 6 mercaptopurine	Promotes oxidation-antioxidation balance and prevents myocardial injury caused by ischemia-reperfusion	
Biological DMARDs TNF antagonist	Regulates leukocyte activation and maturation, cytokine and chemokine release, and reactive oxygen species production.	Promotes cholesterol transport, improves glucose metabolism, downregulates adhesion molecules, and resists the influence of inflammation on blood coagulation, all of which protects the myocardium	May worsen ventricular dysfunction. Thus, it is not recommended for patients with HF
Abatacept	Regulator of the costimulatory signal of T-cell activation and affects the endothelial function	The risk of CVD is 20% less in comparison to using TNF	Consider in patients with established CVD

(Continued)

Table 12.1 (Continued) Autoimmune rheumatic disease medications and cardiovascular effects

| Class | Medication | | | |
	Name	MOA	CVD effect	Prevention
	Rituximab	Anti-CD20 antibody	Anti-CD20-mediated B-cell depletion has been shown to reduce plaque burden in vitro	Can cause peripheral edema, hypertension, hypotension, or arrhythmia. Thus, avoid in patients with these findings at baseline
	Tocilizumab	IL-6 Inhibitor	Atherosclerosis inhibiting effects	
	Anakinra	IL-1 receptor antagonist	Improves cardiac remodeling post-MI without increasing the risk of HF	
Targeted synthesis DMARDs	Tofacitinib and Baricitinib	JAK Inhibitors	Potential increased risk of developing thromboembolic events	Patients prone to thromboembolic events with risk factors like age ≥50 years, smoking, hormonal therapy, and history of thromboembolism should avoid this medication

Abbreviations: NSAIDs: Non-steroidal anti-inflammatory drugs, MOA: Mechanism of action, CVD: Cardiovascular disease, DMARDs: Disease-modifying antirheumatic drug, TNF: Tumor necrosis factor, JAK: Janus kinase; RR: relative risk.

CARDIO-RHEUMATOLOGY COLLABORATION

One of the important aspects in preventing ASCVD in this population is the collaboration between the experts in those two fields. Patients with autoimmune diseases are now less likely to die from the disease itself but from the comorbid conditions. The emerging cardio-rheumatology field allows these two disciplines to collaborate in risk stratification and optimization of preventive strategies and drug therapies in patients with ARDs. Whether by early screening by the rheumatologist or early referral to the cardiologist, it's important to initiate risk assessment as soon as patients are diagnosed with an ARD. Cardio-rheumatology, an emerging cardiology subspecialty, enables cardiologists to work collaboratively with the rheumatologist to address the systemic inflammation, monitor cardio-specific side effects to medical treatments, and aggressively screen and treat cardiovascular risk factors in patients with ARDs.

LIMITATIONS AND BARRIERS TO ASCVD PREVENTION

Despite the evidence of a higher prevalence of ASCVD in ARDs patients, there continues to be an underestimation of CVD burden (see Table 12.2). This stems from a combination of factors: lack of awareness in patients of their increased risk, lack of screening for CVD in these patients by healthcare providers, inadequate screening tools when screening is performed, and a gap in treatment despite being screened. Moreover, there is limited research specific to patients with ARDs and CVD in general. Most studies examine the association between CVD and rheumatologic disease through retrospective or observational methods, leading to limited data on prospective interventions. Ultimately, this results in a lack of focus on the prevention of ASCVD, undertreatment of cardiovascular risk factors, and a higher risk of premature CVD in patients with chronic inflammatory disease.

There is a low level of awareness amongst patients with rheumatologic disease regarding their increased CVD risk. A systematic literature review revealed that 73–97% of patients were

Table 12.2 Limitations to CVD prevention in autoimmune rheumatic diseases and potential solutions

Limitations

- Low awareness of the increased risk for CVD in patients with autoimmune rheumatic diseases and healthcare providers
- Inadequate screening tools for cardiovascular risk assessment
- Delayed or lack of treatment of CVD

Potential solutions

- Use of disease-specific calculators for risk assessment
- Addition of imaging modalities to further evaluate CVD risk
- Dual cardio-rheumatology clinics with collaboration with primary care providers
- Patient education programs to improve patient self-advocacy

Abbreviation: CVD: Cardiovascular disease.

unaware of an increased risk for CVD, and those with the highest risk for CVD reported low awareness of the comorbidity. Furthermore, another survey revealed that while all rheumatologists were aware of the heightened cardiovascular risk, nearly half of patients and their primary care providers were uninformed regarding the increased risk. A different study in the UK showed that patients with diabetes were up to 12 times as likely to have received vascular screening when compared to patients with RA. Lastly, a cross-sectional study showed that out of a cohort of >300 people with inflammatory arthritis, about 50% of patients were eligible for the initiation of statin therapy but were not on it. This shows that even when available, primary and secondary ASCVD tools are not utilized appropriately.

CONCLUSION

The collaboration among primary care providers, rheumatologists, and preventive cardiologists is the key to reducing the burden of CVD in this population. Such multidisciplinary teams can help alleviate the gaps in management. Improving the communication between primary care providers and rheumatologists can also help highlight the importance of routine cardiac screening that can

ASCVD PRIMARY PREVENTION

Exercise:
All AIRD patients should partake in 150 min/week of moderate intensity or 75 min/week of vigorous intensity aerobic exercise

Diet:
Diets high in fibre, fruit and vegetable intake and low in simple sugars and salt are recommended

Smoking cessation:
All patients should be counseled on smoking cessation

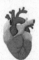

Lipid-lowering therapy
All AIRD patients age 40–75 with a history of diabetes or LDL > 190 mg/dL or ASCVD Risk >20% should initiate statin therapy

ASCVD Risk <20%
<5% "Low Risk"
Emphasize lifestyle to reduce risk factors
5% – <7.5% "Borderline Risk"
Discuss starting statin with patient
7.5% – <20% "Intermediate Risk"
Favors statin therapy especially in RA, SLE & PsA

Other ASCVD Risk Enhancers to consider:
family history of premature ASCVD, persistently elevated LDL-C ≥160 mg/dL, CKD, Metabolic syndrome, Preeclampsia, Premature menopause, HIV, Ethnicity factors (e.g. South Asian ancestory), persistently elevated triglycerides (≥175 mg/mL), hs-CRP ≥2.0 mg/L, Lp(a) levels >50 mg/dL or >125 nmol/L, apoB ≥130 mg/dL, Ankle-brachial index (ABI) <0.9

If risk decision is uncertain:
Consider measuring CAC in selected adults:
CAC = 0 consider no statin (unless diabetes, family history of premature CHD, or cigarette smoking are present)
CAC = 1–99 favors statin (especially after age 55)
CAC = 100+ and/or ≥75th percentile, initiate statin therapy

Anti-hypertensive therapy:
All AIRD patients with an SBP > 130 mmHg or DBP > 80 mmHg should be initiated on anti-hypertensive therapy with either: ACEi/ARB, CCB, or thiazide

Glycemic therapy:
All AIRD patients with T2DM are recommended to start a GLP-1 agonist and/or an SGLT-2 inhibitor

Figure 12.1 Primary ASCVD prevention in rheumatologic diseases.

ASCVD SECONDARY PREVENTION

Exercise:
All AIRD patients should partake in 150 min/week of moderate intensity or 75 min/week of vigorous intensity aerobic exercise
Cardiac Rehab is recommended for rheumatologic patients with angina, heart failure or after MI or revascularization

Diet:
Diets high in fibre, fruit and vegetable intake and low in simple sugars and salt are recommended.

Smoking cessation:
All patients should be counseled on smoking cessation

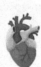

Lipid-lowering Therapy:
All rheumatologic patients with clinical ASCVD should initiate statin therapy for LDL reduction >50% with a goal LDL < 70
If LDL > 70 mg/dl on maximal intensity statin, consider addition of ezemetimibe
If LDL > 70 mg/dl on statin + ezetimibe consider addition of PSK-9 inhibitor

Antiplatelet therapy:
All rheumatologic patients with clinical ASCVD should take Aspirin 81 mg daily
After ACS, PCI dual-antiplatelet therapy should be initiated for approximately 12 months

Anti-hypertensive therapy:
All rheumatologic patients with clinical ASCVD and a SBP > 130 mmHg or DBP > 80 mmHg should be initiated on anti-hypertensive therapy with either: ACEi/ARB, CCB, or thiazide

Glycemic therapy:
All rheumatologic patients with T2DM are recommended to start a GLP-1 agonist and/or an SGLT-2 inhibitor with an HbA1c goal <7%

Figure 12.2 Secondary ASCVD prevention in rheumatologic diseases.

be done by the PCP, while cardio-rheumatology clinics provide an opportunity to prioritize management without taking away from the time dedicated to standard preventative health screenings or necessary rheumatology follow ups.

TAKE-HOME POINTS

- ARDs are systemic inflammatory diseases that affect the cardiovascular system in varying degrees, including the vasculature, myocardium, pericardium, valves, and the conduction system, which can present silently or lead to critical conditions with high morbidity and mortality.

- Traditional and non-traditional disease-specific risk factors contribute to ASCVD in the ARD population.
- Primary and secondary ASCVD preventions include risk-prediction scores, biomarkers, and imaging techniques, as well as the choice of ARD medication.
- The emerging cardio-rheumatology field allows these two disciplines to collaborate in risk stratification and optimization of preventive strategies and drug therapies in patients with ARDs.
- There are many barriers and limitations to ASCVD prevention in ARDs, including but not limited to inadequate or delayed screening, undertreatment of traditional risk factors, not taking into consideration ASCVD in burden management planning, and risk underestimation, as well as a lack of awareness with varying health literacy levels on the patients' end.

REFERENCES

1. Akin I, Nienaber CA. "Obesity paradox" in coronary artery disease. *World J Cardiol.* 2015;7(10):603–608.
2. Alhusain A, Bruce IN. Cardiovascular risk and inflammatory rheumatic diseases. *Clin Med (Lond).* 2013;13(4):395–397.
3. Alenghat FJ. The prevalence of atherosclerosis in those with inflammatory connective tissue disease by race, age, and traditional risk factors. *Sci Rep.* 2016;6:20303.
4. Arnett DK, Blumenthal RS, Albert MA, et al. 2019 ACC/AHA guideline on the primary prevention of cardiovascular disease: a report of the American College of Cardiology/American Heart Association task force on clinical practice guidelines. *Circulation.* 2019;140(11):e596–e646.
5. Arora A, Ingle V, Joshi R, Malik R, Khandelwal G. Exploring the subclinical atherosclerotic load in patients with rheumatoid arthritis: a cross-sectional study. *Cureus.* 2022;14(12):e32644.
6. Atzeni F, Corda M, Gianturco L, Porcu M, Sarzi-Puttini P, Turiel M. Cardiovascular imaging techniques in systemic rheumatic diseases. *Front Med (Lausanne).* 2018;5:26.
7. Atzeni F, Turiel M, Caporali R, et al. The effect of pharmacological therapy on the cardiovascular system of patients with systemic rheumatic diseases. *Autoimmun Rev.* 2010;9(12):835–839.
8. Au K, Singh MK, Bodukam V, et al. Atherosclerosis in systemic sclerosis: a systematic review and meta-analysis. *Arthritis Rheum.* 2011;63(7):2078–2090.
9. Aviña-Zubieta JA, Choi HK, Sadatsafavi M, Etminan M, Esdaile JM, Lacaille D. Risk of cardiovascular mortality in patients with rheumatoid arthritis: a meta-analysis of observational studies. *Arthritis Rheum.* 2008;59(12):1690–1697.
10. Baoqi Y, Dan M, Xingxing Z, et al. Effect of anti-rheumatic drugs on cardiovascular disease events in rheumatoid arthritis. *Front Cardiovasc Med.* 2021;8:812631.
11. Bartels CM, Roberts TJ, Hansen KE, et al. Rheumatologist and primary care management of cardiovascular disease risk in rheumatoid arthritis: patient and provider perspectives. *Arthritis Care Res (Hoboken).* 2016;68(4):415–423.
12. Bartoloni E, Alunno A, Bistoni O, Gerli R. Cardiovascular risk in rheumatoid arthritis and systemic autoimmune rheumatic disorders: a suggested model of preventive strategy. *Clin Rev Allergy Immunol.* 2013;44(1):14–22.
13. Bettiol A, Alibaz-Oner F, Direskeneli H, et al. Vascular Behçet syndrome: from pathogenesis to treatment. *Nat Rev Rheumatol.* 2023;19(2):111–126.
14. Brevetti G, Giugliano G, Brevetti L, Hiatt WR. Inflammation in peripheral artery disease. *Circulation.* 2010;122(18):1862–1875.
15. Borba EF, Bonfá E. Dyslipoproteinemias in systemic lupus erythematosus: influence of disease, activity, and anticardiolipin antibodies. *Lupus.* 1997;6(6):533–539.
16. Borg FA, Dasgupta B. Peripheral arterial disease in polymyalgia rheumatica. *Arthritis Res Ther.* 2009;11(3):111.

17. Cai W, Tang X, Pang M. Prevalence of metabolic syndrome in patients with rheumatoid arthritis: an updated systematic review and meta-analysis. *Front Med (Lausanne)*. 2022;9:855141.

18. Champion HC. The heart in scleroderma. *Rheum Dis Clin North Am*. 2008;34(1): 181–190; viii.

19. Chen DY, Sawamura T, Dixon RAF, Sánchez-Quesada JL, Chen CH. Autoimmune rheumatic diseases: an update on the role of atherogenic electronegative LDL and potential therapeutic strategies. *J Clin Med*. 2021;10(9):1992.

20. Chung CP, Oeser A, Solus JF, et al. Inflammation-associated insulin resistance: differential effects in rheumatoid arthritis and systemic lupus erythematosus define potential mechanisms. *Arthritis Rheum*. 2008;58(7):2105–2112.

21. Colantonio LD, Hubbard D, Monda KL, et al. Atherosclerotic risk and statin use among patients with peripheral artery disease. *J Am Coll Cardiol*. 2020;76(3):251–264.

22. Cottin Y, Issa R, Benalia M, et al. Association between serum osteoprotegerin levels and severity of coronary artery disease in patients with acute myocardial infarction. *J Clin Med*. 2021;10(19):4326.

23. Coutinho M, Gerstein HC, Wang Y, Yusuf S. The relationship between glucose and incident cardiovascular events. A metaregression analysis of published data from 20 studies of 95,783 individuals followed for 12.4 years. *Diabetes Care*. 1999;22(2):233–240.

24. Crowson CS, Myasoedova E, Davis JM, et al. Use of B-type natriuretic peptide as a screening tool for left ventricular diastolic dysfunction in rheumatoid arthritis patients without clinical cardiovascular disease. *Arthritis Care Res (Hoboken)*. 2011;63(5):729–734.

25. Desai CS, Lee DC, Shah SJ. Systemic sclerosis and the heart: current diagnosis and management. *Curr Opin Rheumatol*. 2011;23(6):545–554.

26. Dhakal BP, Kim CH, Al-Kindi SG, Oliveira GH. Heart failure in systemic lupus erythematosus. *Trends Cardiovasc Med*. 2018;28(3):187–197.

27. Durante A, Bronzato S. The increased cardiovascular risk in patients affected by autoimmune diseases: review of the various manifestations. *J Clin Med Res*. 2015;7(6):379–384.

28. Ferhatbegović L, Mršić D, Kušljugić S, Pojskić B. LDL-C: the only causal risk factor for ASCVD. Why is it still overlooked and underestimated? *Curr Atheroscler Rep*. 2022;24(8):635–642.

29. Frostegård J. Atherosclerosis in patients with autoimmune disorders. *Arterioscler Thromb Vasc Biol*. 2005;25(9):1776–1785.

30. Gallucci G, Tartarone A, Lerose R, Lalinga AV, Capobianco AM. Cardiovascular risk of smoking and benefits of smoking cessation. *J Thorac Dis*. 2020;12(7):3866–3876.

31. Gelfand JM, Neimann AL, Shin DB, Wang X, Margolis DJ, Troxel AB. Risk of myocardial infarction in patients with psoriasis. *JAMA*. 2006;296(14):1735–1741.

32. Geovanini GR, Libby P. Atherosclerosis and inflammation: overview and updates. *Clin Sci (Lond)*. 2018;132(12):1243–1252.

33. Ghosh-Swaby OR, Kuriya B. Awareness and perceived risk of cardiovascular disease among individuals living with rheumatoid arthritis is low: results of a systematic literature review. *Arthritis Res Ther*. 2019;21(1):33. doi:10.1186/s13075-019-1817-y

34. Greenland P, Blaha MJ, Budoff MJ, Erbel R, Watson KE. Coronary calcium score and cardiovascular risk. *J Am Coll Cardiol*. 2018;72(4):434–447. doi:10.1016/j.jacc.2018.05.027

35. Heidenreich PA, Bozkurt B, Aguilar D, et al. 2022 AHA/ACC/HFSA guideline for the management of heart failure: executive summary: a report of the American College of Cardiology/American Heart Association joint committee on clinical practice guidelines. *Circulation*. 2022;145(18):e876–e894. doi:10.1161/CIR.0000000000001062

36. Han C, Robinson DW, Hackett MV, Paramore LC, Fraeman KH, Bala MV. Cardiovascular disease and risk factors in patients with rheumatoid arthritis, psoriatic arthritis, and ankylosing spondylitis. *J Rheumatol*. 2006;33(11):2167–2172.

37. Hill MF, Bordoni B. *Hyperlipidemia*. 2023.

38. Ho JSY, Rohra V, Korb L, Perera B. Cardiovascular risk quantification using QRISK-3 score in people with intellectual disability. *BJPsych Open*. 2021;7(S1):S52–S53. doi:10.1192/bjo.2021.187

39. Hollan I, Meroni PL, Ahearn JM, et al. Cardiovascular disease in autoimmune rheumatic diseases. *Autoimmun Rev*. 2013;12(10):1004–1015. doi:10.1016/j.autrev.2013.03.013

40. Hon KL, Leung AKC. Neonatal lupus erythematosus. *Autoimmune Dis*. 2012;2012:301274. doi:10.1155/2012/301274

41. Huang S, Cai T, Weber BN, et al. Association between inflammation, incident heart failure, and heart failure subtypes in patients with rheumatoid arthritis. *Arthritis Care Res (Hoboken)*. 2023;75(5):1036–1045. doi:10.1002/acr.24804

42. Jain A, McClelland RL, Polak JF, et al. Cardiovascular imaging for assessing cardiovascular risk in asymptomatic men versus women. *Circ Cardiovasc Imaging*. 2011;4(1):8–15. doi:10.1161/CIRCIMAGING.110.959403

43. Jesson C, Bohbot Y, Soudet S, et al. Is the calcium score useful for rheumatoid arthritis patients at low or intermediate cardiovascular risk? *J Clin Med*. 2022;11(16):4841. doi:10.3390/jcm11164841

44. Katz G, Smilowitz NR, Blazer A, Clancy R, Buyon JP, Berger JS. Systemic lupus erythematosus and increased prevalence of atherosclerotic cardiovascular disease in hospitalized patients. *Mayo Clin Proc*. 2019;94(8):1436–1443. doi:10.1016/j.mayocp.2019.01.044

45. Kelsey MD, Nelson AJ, Green JB, et al. Guidelines for cardiovascular risk reduction in patients with type 2 diabetes: JACC guideline comparison. *J Am Coll Cardiol*. 2022;79(18):1849–1857. doi:10.1016/j.jacc.2022.02.046

46. Kerola AM, Rollefstad S, Semb AG. Atherosclerotic cardiovascular disease in rheumatoid arthritis: impact of inflammation and antirheumatic treatment. *Eur Cardiol*. 2021;16:e18. doi:10.15420/ecr.2020.44

47. Kremers HM, Nicola PJ, Crowson CS, Ballman KV, Gabriel SE. Prognostic importance of low body mass index in relation to cardiovascular mortality in rheumatoid arthritis. *Arthritis Rheum*. 2004;50(11):3450–3457. doi:10.1002/art.20612

48. Kumar N, Armstrong DJ. Cardiovascular disease–the silent killer in rheumatoid arthritis. *Clin Med (Lond)*. 2008;8(4):384–387. doi:10.7861/clinmedicine.8-4-384

49. Kuriya B, Akhtari S, Movahedi M, et al. Statin use for primary cardiovascular disease prevention is low in inflammatory arthritis. *Can J Cardiol*. 2022;38(8):1244–1252. doi:10.1016/j.cjca.2022.04.002

50. Lambova S. Cardiac manifestations in systemic sclerosis. *World J Cardiol*. 2014;6(9):993–1005. doi:10.4330/wjc.v6.i9.993

51. Leung N, Fang C, Pendse J, Toprover M, Pillinger MH. Narrative review: peripheral arterial disease in patients with hyperuricemia and gout. *Curr Rheumatol Rep*. 2023;25(5):83–97. doi:10.1007/s11926-023-01100-1

52. López-Mejías R, Corrales A, Genre F, et al. Angiopoietin-2 serum levels correlate with severity, early onset and cardiovascular disease in patients with rheumatoid arthritis. *Clin Exp Rheumatol*. 2013;31(5):761–766.

53. López-Mejias R, Ubilla B, Genre F, et al. Osteoprotegerin concentrations relate independently to established cardiovascular disease in rheumatoid arthritis. *J Rheumatol*. 2015;42(1):39–45. doi:10.3899/jrheum.140690

54. Martinez-Moreno A, Ocampo-Candiani J, Garza-Rodriguez V. Psoriasis and cardiovascular disease: a narrative review. *Korean J Fam Med*. 2021;42(5):345–355. doi:10.4082/kjfm.20.0053

55. McMahon M, Hahn BH, Skaggs BJ. Systemic lupus erythematosus and cardiovascular disease: prediction and potential for therapeutic intervention. *Expert Rev Clin Immunol*. 2011;7(2):227–241. doi:10.1586/eci.10.98

56. Miller ER, Pastor-Barriuso R, Dalal D, Riemersma RA, Appel LJ, Guallar E. Meta-analysis: high-dosage vitamin E supplementation may increase all-cause mortality. *Ann Intern Med*. 2005;142(1):37. doi:10.7326/0003-4819-142-1-200501040-00110

57. Mills KT, Stefanescu A, He J. The global epidemiology of hypertension. *Nat Rev Nephrol*. 2020;16(4):223–237. doi:10.1038/s41581-019-0244-2

58. Monk HL, Muller S, Mallen CD, Hider SL. Cardiovascular screening in rheumatoid arthritis: a cross-sectional primary care database study. *BMC Fam Pract*. 2013;14:150. doi:10.1186/1471-2296-14-150

59. Moran CA, Collins LF, Beydoun N, et al. Cardiovascular implications of immune disorders in women. *Circ Res*. 2022;130(4):593–610. doi:10.1161/CIRCRESAHA.121.319877

60. Mortensen MB, Blaha MJ. Is there a role of coronary CTA in primary prevention? Current state and future directions. *Curr Atheroscler Rep*. 2021;23(8):44. doi:10.1007/s11883-021-00943-2

61. Nicola PJ, Maradit-Kremers H, Roger VL, et al. The risk of congestive heart failure in rheumatoid arthritis: a population-based study over 46 years. *Arthritis Rheum*. 2005;52(2):412–420. doi:10.1002/art.20855

62. Ninomiya T, Perkovic V, de Galan BE, et al. Albuminuria and kidney function independently predict cardiovascular and renal outcomes in diabetes. *J Am Soc Nephrol*. 2009;20(8):1813–1821. doi:10.1681/ASN.2008121270

63. Nissen SE, Yeomans ND, Solomon DH, et al. Cardiovascular safety of celecoxib, naproxen, or ibuprofen for arthritis. *N Engl J Med*. 2016;375(26):2519–2529. doi:10.1056/NEJMoa1611593

64. Patel J, Al Rifai M, Scheuner MT, et al. Basic vs more complex definitions of family history in the prediction of coronary heart disease: the multi-ethnic study of atherosclerosis. *Mayo Clin Proc*. 2018;93(9):1213–1223. doi:10.1016/j.mayocp.2018.01.014

65. Prasad M, Hermann J, Gabriel SE, et al. Cardiorheumatology: cardiac involvement in systemic rheumatic disease. *Nat Rev Cardiol*. 2015;12(3):168–176. doi:10.1038/nrcardio.2014.206

66. Quesada O, Lauzon M, Buttle R, et al. Body weight and physical fitness in women with ischaemic heart disease: does physical fitness contribute to our understanding of the obesity paradox in women? *Eur J Prev Cardiol*. 2022;29(12):1608–1614. doi:10.1093/eurjpc/zwac046

67. Petri M, Lakatta C, Magder L, Goldman D. Effect of prednisone and hydroxychloroquine on coronary artery disease risk factors in systemic lupus erythematosus: a longitudinal data analysis. *Am J Med*. 1994;96(3):254–259. doi:10.1016/0002-9343(94)90151-1

68. Peters MJL, Symmons DPM, McCarey D, et al. EULAR evidence-based recommendations for cardiovascular risk management in patients with rheumatoid arthritis and other forms of inflammatory arthritis. *Ann Rheum Dis*. 2010;69(2):325–331. doi:10.1136/ard.2009.113696

69. Pinto AJ, Roschel H, de Sá Pinto AL, et al. Physical inactivity and sedentary behavior: overlooked risk factors in autoimmune rheumatic diseases? *Autoimmun Rev*. 2017;16(7):667–674. doi:10.1016/j.autrev.2017.05.001

70. Reiss AB, Carsons SE, Anwar K, et al. Atheroprotective effects of methotrexate on reverse cholesterol transport proteins and foam cell transformation in human THP-1 monocyte/macrophages. *Arthritis Rheum*. 2008;58(12):3675–3683. doi:10.1002/art.24040

71. Ridker PM, MacFadyen JG, Glynn RJ, Bradwin G, Hasan AA, Rifai N. Comparison of interleukin-6, C-reactive protein, and low-density lipoprotein cholesterol as biomarkers of residual risk in contemporary practice: secondary analyses from the cardiovascular inflammation reduction trial. *Eur Heart J*. 2020;41(31):2952–2961. doi:10.1093/eurheartj/ehaa160

72. Roldan CA, Chavez J, Wiest PW, Qualls CR, Crawford MH. Aortic root disease and valve disease associated with ankylosing spondylitis. *J Am Coll Cardiol*. 1998;32(5):1397–1404. doi:10.1016/s0735-1097(98)00393-3

73. Roman MJ, Salmon JE. Cardiovascular manifestations of rheumatologic diseases. *Circulation*. 2007;116(20):2346–2355. doi:10.1161/CIRCULATIONAHA.106.678334

74. Roncaglioni MC, Santoro L, D'Avanzo B, et al. Role of family history in patients with myocardial infarction. An Italian case-control study. GISSI-EFRIM Investigators. *Circulation*. 1992;85(6):2065–2072. doi:10.1161/01.cir.85.6.2065

75. Ross R. Atherosclerosis–an inflammatory disease. *N Engl J Med*. 1999;340(2):115–126. doi:10.1056/NEJM199901143400207

76. Rozanski A, Blumenthal JA, Kaplan J. Impact of psychological factors on the pathogenesis of cardiovascular disease and implications for therapy. *Circulation*. 1999;99(16):2192–2217. doi:10.1161/01.cir.99.16.2192

77. Rudolf H, Mügge A, Trampisch HJ, Scharnagl H, März W, Kara K. NT-proBNP for risk prediction of cardiovascular events and all-cause mortality: the getABI-study. *Int J Cardiol Heart Vasc*. 2020;29:100553. doi:10.1016/j.ijcha.2020.100553

78. Sagonas I, Daoussis D. Serotonin and systemic sclerosis. An emerging player in pathogenesis. *Joint Bone Spine*. 2022;89(3):105309. doi:10.1016/j.jbspin.2021.105309

79. Schäfer C, Keyßer G. Lifestyle factors and their influence on rheumatoid arthritis: a narrative review. *J Clin Med*. 2022;11(23):7179. doi:10.3390/jcm11237179

80. Seferović PM, Ristić AD, Maksimović R, et al. Cardiac arrhythmias and conduction disturbances in autoimmune rheumatic diseases. *Rheumatology (Oxford)*. 2006;45 Suppl 4:iv39–42. doi:10.1093/rheumatology/kel315

81. Sharif K, Watad A, Bragazzi NL, Lichtbroun M, Amital H, Shoenfeld Y. Physical activity and autoimmune diseases: get moving and manage the disease. *Autoimmun Rev*. 2018;17(1):53–72. doi:10.1016/j.autrev.2017.11.010

82. Sherer Y, Shoenfeld Y. Mechanisms of disease: atherosclerosis in autoimmune diseases. *Nat Clin Pract Rheumatol*. 2006;2(2):99–106. doi:10.1038/ncprheum0092

83. Solomon DH, Karlson EW, Rimm EB, et al. Cardiovascular morbidity and mortality in women diagnosed with rheumatoid arthritis. *Circulation*. 2003;107(9):1303–1307. doi:10.1161/01.cir.0000054612.26458.b2

84. Su D, Li Z, Li X, et al. Association between serum interleukin-6 concentration and mortality in patients with coronary artery disease. *Mediators Inflamm*. 2013;2013:1–7. doi:10.1155/2013/726178

85. Symmons DPM, Gabriel SE. Epidemiology of CVD in rheumatic disease, with a focus on RA and SLE. *Nat Rev Rheumatol*. 2011;7(7):399–408. doi:10.1038/nrrheum.2011.75

86. Udachkina HV, Novikova DS, Popkova TV, et al. Calcification of coronary arteries in early rheumatoid arthritis prior to anti-rheumatic therapy. *Rheumatol Int*. 2018;38(2):211–217. doi:10.1007/s00296-017-3860-9

87. van Sijl AM, Peters MJ, Knol DK, et al. Carotid intima media thickness in rheumatoid arthritis as compared to control subjects: a meta-analysis. *Semin Arthritis Rheum*. 2011;40(5):389–397. doi:10.1016/j.semarthrit.2010.06.006

88. Virani SS, Alonso A, Benjamin EJ, et al. Heart disease and stroke statistics-2020 update: a report from the American Heart Association. *Circulation*. 2020;141(9):e139–e596. doi:10.1161/CIR.0000000000000757

89. Wasko MCM, Hubert HB, Lingala VB, et al. Hydroxychloroquine and risk of diabetes in patients with rheumatoid arthritis. *JAMA*. 2007;298(2):187. doi:10.1001/jama.298.2.187

90. Watson DJ, Rhodes T, Guess HA. All-cause mortality and vascular events among patients with rheumatoid arthritis, osteoarthritis, or no arthritis in the UK general practice research database. *J Rheumatol*. 2003;30(6):1196–1202.

91. WHO. Prevalence of small vessel and large vessel disease in diabetic patients from 14 centres. The world health organisation multinational study of vascular disease in diabetics. Diabetes drafting group. *Diabetologia*. 1985;28(Suppl):615–640. doi:10.1007/BF00290267

92. Williams JN, Drenkard C, Lim SS. The impact of social determinants of health on the presentation, management and outcomes of systemic lupus erythematosus. *Rheumatology (Oxford)*. 2023;62(Suppl 1): i10–i14.

93. Willerson JT, Ridker PM. Inflammation as a cardiovascular risk factor. *Circulation*. 2004;109(21 Suppl 1):II2–10.

94. Wilson PWF, Bozeman SR, Burton TM, Hoaglin DC, Ben-Joseph R, Pashos CL. Prediction of first events of coronary heart disease and stroke with consideration of adiposity. *Circulation*. 2008;118(2):124–130.

95. Wisłowska M, Sypuła S, Kowalik I. Echocardiographic findings and 24-h electrocardiographic Holter monitoring in patients with nodular and non-nodular rheumatoid arthritis. *Rheumatol Int*. 1999;18(5–6):163–169.

13

Future directions for cardio-rheumatology

C. NOEL BAIREY MERZ, JANET WEI, AND MARTHA GULATI
Disclosure: C. Noel Bairey Merz – iRhythm, SHL Telemedicine

INTRODUCTION

Patients with inflammatory rheumatic diseases have an increased risk of cardiovascular disease (CVD) in comparison to the general population.[1] The higher CVD in patients with rheumatic diseases is not sufficiently explained by differences in the prevalence of traditional CVD factors.[2–5] Chronic inflammation has been considered a key feature in CVD pathogenesis in rheumatologic diseases.[6] Conversely, patients with RMDs are often exposed to immunomodulators and glucocorticoids. However, better control of inflammation (e.g., immunomodulators and glucocorticoids) may reduce CVD in individual patients.[7,8] An important knowledge gap exists regarding if the side effects of rheumatologic medications outweigh any anti-inflammatory benefit, thereby increasing the CVD.

Clinical trials have established that inflammation participates causally in human atherosclerosis.[9] This suggests novel anti-inflammatory treatments that add to established therapies to help stem the growing global epidemic of CVD. Indeed, a number of potential treatment targets are being tested in CVD to optimize beneficial effects and avoid interference with host defenses or other unwanted actions.[10] This "inflammation" intersection between rheumatologic disease and CVD is an area to investigate for improved risk detection, prevention, and management of CVD in rheumatologic disease.

CURRENT STATUS

The majority of rheumatologic diseases are uncommon, therefore limiting the ability to perform large observational studies to assess the impact of traditional and disease-specific risk factors on CVD burden and clinical trials on the long-term cardiovascular effects of preventive treatments.[11] This small cohort size limits the generation of Class I evidence-based guidelines that typically require randomized, controlled clinical trials. Investigation of therapies that are confounded by indication is a common limitation in many observational studies. This leaves practitioners to rely on expert opinion and consensus documents. There is a clear need for future studies to identify exposures and outcomes more rigorously to overcome these methodological issues.

The current methods of CVD risk assessment are controversial. Only a few guidelines recommend the use of formal risk calculators. These are the EULAR guidelines suggesting the use of SCORE and the British Society for Rheumatology guidelines performed in collaboration with NICE, preferring the use of QRISK-2.[12] A focus on risk calculators developed for the general population taking into account rheumatologic disease or rheumatologic-specific risk calculators, such as the Expanded Cardiovascular Risk Prediction Score for rheumatoid arthritis, is currently proposed.[12]

DOI: 10.1201/9781003386711-13

FUTURE DIRECTIONS

Future research for improving CVD management in rheumatic and musculoskeletal diseases has been summarized by European League Against Rheumatism (EULAR) multidisciplinary task force and summarized in Table 13.1.[11]

Specifically, individual patient clinical phenotype for CVD risk assessment and cardiovascular prognosis also merits further investigation. One of the challenges is the better identification of patient subgroups at higher CVD risk, including, for example, those with longer disease duration and a number of flares/relapses (or those with certain demographic and disease characteristics).

Table 13.1 Research agenda and future perspectives

1. Validation of existing generic and modified CVD prediction tools in large prospective studies, and development of new disease-specific equations.
2. Additive value of vascular imaging and/or circulating biomarkers in CVD assessment in RMDs.
3. Identification of patient subgroups with higher CVD.
4. Long-term effects of current and new drugs for rheumatologic diseases on CVD factors and cardiovascular events.
5. Role of antithrombotic agents used in some rheumatologic diseases (e.g., aspirin, LMWH in SLE/APS) to reduce the overall CVD in these patients.
6. Need for large educational campaigns within the rheumatological and other medical specialties and patient associations to increase CVD awareness.
7. Best implementation methods for the CVD recommendations.

Abbreviations: APS, antiphospholipid syndrome; CVD, cardiovascular disease; LMWH, low-molecular weight heparin; RMDs, rheumatic and musculoskeletal diseases; SLE, systemic lupus erythematosus.

Source: Reprinted with permission EULAR recommendations for cardiovascular risk management in rheumatic and musculoskeletal diseases, including systemic lupus erythematosus and antiphospholipid syndrome | Annals of the Rheumatic Diseases (bmj.com)

Long-term effects of current and new drugs for rheumatologic diseases on CVD need further investigation. Several anti-inflammatory agents (e.g., colchicine, anti-IL1b) have been shown to lower cardiovascular outcomes in randomized controlled trials for secondary prevention of CVD in the general population, and other trials are ongoing (e.g., hydroxychloroquine), but further evidence is needed on the cardiovascular outcomes and safety of such immunoregulatory agents in rheumatologic diseases.[13,14] More evidence is needed about the effect of glucocorticoids, NSAIDs, and IL-1 antagonists, the dosage and duration of colchicine treatment, and the risk and benefits of the concomitant use of colchicine and statins in patients with gout.

Sodium-glucose co-transporter 2 inhibitors (SGLT2i, dapagliflozin, canagliflozin, and empagliflozin) are a class of oral hypoglycemic medication for the management of Type II diabetes mellitus (T2D); they have also been demonstrated to lead to weight loss, decrease atherosclerotic cardiovascular risk, improve heart failure, reduce proteinuria, and prevent progression to end-stage renal disease (ESRD) in patients with chronic kidney disease. SGLT2i could have multiple benefits for patients with rheumatic diseases; however, these patients have not been included in clinical trials. A recent observational study suggests increased prescribing in rheumatic diseases.[15] Future work should be directed in this area.

REFERENCES

1. England BR, Thiele GM, Anderson DR, Mikuls TR. Increased cardiovascular risk in rheumatoid arthritis: mechanisms and implications. BMJ. 2018;361:k1036.
2. Choi HK, Curhan G. Independent impact of gout on mortality and risk for coronary heart disease. Circulation. 2007;116(8):894–900.
3. Clarson LE, et al. Increased risk of vascular disease associated with gout: a retrospective, matched cohort study in the UK clinical practice research datalink. Ann Rheum Dis. 2015;74(4):642–7.
4. Kurmann RD, et al. Cardiovascular risk factors and atherosclerotic cardiovascular events among incident cases of systemic

sclerosis: results from a population-based cohort (1980-2016). Mayo Clin Proc. 2020;95(7):1369–78.

5. Geovanini GR, Libby P. Atherosclerosis and inflammation: overview and updates. Clin Sci (Lond). 2018;132(12):1243–52.

6. Manzi S, Wasko MC. Inflammation-mediated rheumatic diseases and atherosclerosis. Ann Rheum Dis. 2000;59(5):321–5.

7. Ajala ON, Everett BM. Targeting inflammation to reduce residual cardiovascular risk. Curr Atheroscler Rep. 2020;22(11):66.

8. Lawler PR, et al. Targeting cardiovascular inflammation: next steps in clinical translation. Eur Heart J. 2021;42(1):113–31.

9. Libby P. The changing landscape of atherosclerosis. Nature. 2021;592(7855):524–33.

10. Libby P. Targeting inflammatory pathways in cardiovascular disease: the inflammasome, interleukin-1, interleukin-6 and beyond. Cells. 2021;10(4):951.

11. Drosos GC, et al. EULAR recommendations for cardiovascular risk management in rheumatic and musculoskeletal diseases, including systemic lupus erythematosus and antiphospholipid syndrome. Ann Rheum Dis. 2022;81(6):768–79.

12. Bonek K, Gluszko P. Cardiovascular risk assessment in rheumatoid arthritis - controversies and the new approach. Reumatologia. 2016;54(3):128–35.

13. Tardif JC, et al. Efficacy and safety of low-dose colchicine after myocardial infarction. N Engl J Med. 2019;381(26):2497–505.

14. Ridker PM, et al. Antiinflammatory therapy with canakinumab for atherosclerotic disease. N Engl J Med. 2017;377(12):1119–31.

15. Oakes EEJ, Choi M, Guan H, Costenbader K. Prescribing patterns of SGLT2 inhibitors for patients with autoimmune rheumatic disease. Arthritis Rheumatol. 2023;74:1472–4.

Index

Note: **Bold** page numbers refer to **tables** and *Italic* page numbers refer to *figures*.

For Product Safety Concerns and Information please contact our EU
representative GPSR@taylorandfrancis.com
Taylor & Francis Verlag GmbH, Kaufingerstraße 24, 80331 München, Germany